NUTRITION FOR VEGETARIANS

by
Agatha Moody Thrash, M.D.
and
Calvin L. Thrash, Jr., M.D.

Nutrition for Vegetarians
By Agatha Moody Thrash, M.D. and
Calvin L. Thrash, Jr. M.D.

A NewLifestyle Book / Updated September, 1996
Corrections/Additions, April, 1998

PRINTED IN THE UNITED STATES OF AMERICA

Original Printing, 1982
Over 100,000 copies in print

2500 September, 1996
5000 April, 1998

ISBN: 0-942658-03-5

NewLifestyle Books
Seale, AL 36875
U.S.A.
334/855-4708
(800) 542-5695

FOREWORD

It is such a privilege to study nutrition. Not only is it an exciting science to trace out, but it shows the great love of a wise and resourceful Creator in providing nourishing and pleasant foods from the elements of the ground for those who were created in His image from these same elements. In the study of nutrition one finds some parts that are purely artistic—that which has to do with colors, odors, flavors, textures, and blends; and also that which has to do with the appreciation of cultural features, and the psychology of food acceptance.

In addition to those features of nutrition there is that which is purely scientific—weights and measures, chemical reactions, observation of function, and such matters. but above all these is the choice gem in the study of nutrition that has to do with moral and religious matters. It is the hope of the authors that this book will enable you to experience the joy of seeing lessons of philosophical value from a study of the physical sciences. "As in the physical, so in the spiritual." NUTRITION FOR VEGETARIANS is designed to present more to the mind than mere facts and figures, but to appeal to the spiritual and esthetic as well.

In this presentation no attempt has been made to cover completely any phase of nutrition. Rather those topics have been explored that are of particular interest to the authors and to those who follow a vegetarian diet. A large part of what is presented is a result of our search to insure the most favorable diet for the growth and development of our two children, Carol Ann and Calvin L. They have grown from preschoolers to young adults without disease, broken bones, or dental cavities. Our major motivating factor in adopting a vegeterian lifestyle was to protect our children and our patients from the many diseases that can be transmitted from animals to humans. When the link between human cancer and the existing reservoir of cancer in the animal kingdom began to be suspected, we felt we would never be able to forgive ourselves if one of our children came down with leukemia or some maiming disease because of their exposure to foods of animal origin. We have found the vegetarian lifestyle one of the rich joys of life, and would surely give this experience the superlative characterization of a grand adventure.

One of the persons who read the rough manuscript wrote the following: "It has been of great benefit to me to read this manuscript....May this book be a partial answer to the cry,

Ho, everyone that thirsteth (for health and salvation)
Come ye to the waters.
And he that hath no money,
Come buy milk (the Word) and wine (the blood)
Without money and without price
Wherefore do you spend your money
For that which is not bread,
Or your labor for that which
Satisfies not.
Harken diligently to Me and delight
Your soul in fatness (abundant health) Isa. 55:1

We trust that you will feel rewarded for having studied the art, the delicate culture, and the science of nutrition for vegetarians.

Agatha M. Thrash, M.D.

FOREWORD

Why another book on nutrition? As practicing vegetarians for nearly twenty years, thirteen or fourteen of which we have used no animal products or nutrition supplements, we have observed a plethora of myths, misconceptions, taboos, and exaggerations regarding the vegetarian and his diet. These misconceptions are by no means limited to the uneducated. And so it seemed to us that a book would be of value that would seek to dispel many of the misconceptions, that would address itself to the peculiar problems and needs of the vegetarian, that would attempt to answer some of the questions that vegetarians and those desiring to adopt this pleasant lifestyle might have, and that would incorporate certain aspects of modern scientific thought and research.

As source material, we have drawn upon standard textbooks of nutrition, pertinent references from medical and nutrition journals, lectures from prominent nutritionists, and from our personal experiences and observations in the practice of medicine over the past two decades. The last eleven years have presented us with the rare privilege of observing directly and serving any medical needs of up to 150 pure vegetarians at any given time at Yuchi Pines Institute, a rural medical missionary training center in Alabama, operated by Seventh-day Adventist laymen. During this time a considerable number of children have been born at Yuchi Pines Institute, none of whom have ever tasted animal products. With this group we have had opportunities that few of our professors or fellow researchers have ever had, and thus we can speak with some authority on most of the subjects covered in this book, not being limited merely to what is read or heard. Finally, we want to acknowledge our dependence upon certain sources that we consider to be divinely inspired on the subject of health and nutrition; that is, the Bible and the writings of Ellen G. White. This remarkable woman, whose nutrition writings are marveled at by eminent nutritionists of our day such as the late Dr. Clive McKay of Cornell, was over a hundred years ahead of her time. We have been unable to detect erroneous concepts in her writings, certainly a strong evidence for divine inspiration in a field so new and so fickle as nutrition.

Obviously, a book this size is not intended to be exhaustive, and yet we would like to cover the basics of good nutrition as well as to fulfill the objectives noted above. We have wanted to produce a book that would be understandable to the average informed and interested non-scientist, while also having sufficient references to interest the scientifically trained individual (who is often woefully inadequate in this particular field). For this group, we hope to have excited enough interest to stimulate further study in available standard texts and literature, and even "hands on" research, both formal and informal in the growing field of nutrition for vegetarians. For both groups, we hope we have presented clear and stimulating reading to interest everyone in a lifetime of intriguing and enjoyable at-the-table "research" in the world of vegetarianism.

Calvin L. Thrash, Jr. M.D.

CONTENTS

Foreword by Agatha M. Thrash, M.D.
Foreword by Calvin L. Thrash, Jr., M.D.

Chapter One: Why Be a Vegetarian 1

Man Naturally a Vegetarian............................1
Cosmetic Reasons for Being a Vegetarian 1
Religious Reasons......................................1
Economic Reasons......................................1
Length of Life Before the Flood 1
An Historically Reliable Diet 2
Health Reasons...2
Vegetarianism Discussed: Nutritional Superiority 3
Aging Process Slower in Vegetarians 5
Some Psychological Effects of Meat Eating 6
Productive Value of a Simple Diet.........................6
Leukemia Incidence Higher in Cattle Country..............8
Breast and Bowel Cancer Less in Vegetarians 8
No Diabetes and Plenty of Good Teeth 8
How to Feed a Hungry World..............................8
How People Become Vegetarians 9

Chapter Two: Nutrition, Longevity and Usefulness 11

Productivity, the Objective of Nutrition....................11
The Basic Food Groups: Historical Considerations 11
Essential Foods..12
Primary Rule of Nutrition................................12
Deterioration of the Earth at the Present...................13
Man Did Eat Angel's Food 14
Human Appetite Hard to Control 14
Meat is Stimulatory, Not Especially Strengthening 15
Eating Animal Products an Extravagance 15
Relish of Meals Surpasses Former Enjoyment.............15
Never Call an Impoverished Diet Health Reform...........16
Lessons from Nature....................................16

Chapter Three: Function of Food and Food Habits 19

Why Do We Eat...19
Malnutrition..19
Function of Food 20
Deficiency Diseases 21
Types of Energy..21
Heat of Specific Dynamic Action.........................22
Food Habits..22
Cooking and Eating—Science and Art 23
Influence of Habits on Purchases 25

Chapter Four: Growth, Processing, Marketing, and Food Storage 27

Causes of Large Variation of Nutrients in Foods 27
Unsubstantiated Claims for Organic Gardening.............28
Use Both Methods—Organic and Non-Organic............29
Processing of Food......................................29
Marketing..30
Autolytic Enzymes 30

Chapter Five: Carbohydrates 33

The Best Fuel for the Body 33
What Are Carbohydrates.................................33
Uses of Carbohydrates 35
Blood Sugar..37
Gluten-free Diet 38
High Fiber Diet 39
Sugar Causes Problems.................................39

Chapter Six: Fats 43

Chemical Composition 43
Triglycerides- Neutral Fats...............................44
Phospholipid 44
Cholesterol 44
Physical and Chemical Properties of Fats..................44
Functions of Fats.......................................46
Fats and Heart Disease 47
Fat-Soluble Vitamins....................................47
Fatty Acid Content of Foods 47
Sterols...48
Bile Salts and Bile Acids.................................49
Fats Related to Sugar 49

Chapter Seven: Proteins 51

Composition of Proteins..................................51
Protein Absorbed More Efficiently in Shortages............52
Are We Eating Too Much Protein? 52
Naming Errors in Nutrition...............................54
Uses of Protein in the Body 54
Daily Requirements of Protein............................55
Nutritive Effect of Foods Near to Pharmacologic Effects.......56
Types of Protein 56
Specific Dynamic Action.................................58
Purine Content of Foods.................................58
Brain Proteins 59

Chapter Eight: Vitamins **61**

The Vital Amines. 61
Uses of Vitamins. 61
Cooking Instructions for Vitamins 62
Causes of Decreased Absorption from the
Gastrointestinal Tract. 62
How the Body Uses Vitamins. 63
Vitamin B-1 (Thiamine). 63
Vitamin B-2 (Riboflavin) 63
Pellagra. 64
Vitamin B-6 (Pyridoxine) 65
Pantothenic Acid and Biotin 65
Vitamin C. 65
Vitamin D. 66
Vitamin E (Tocopherol) 66
Vitamin B-12. 66
Non-Animal Sources of B-12. 67
B-12 Supplements. 67
B-12 Requirements 68
Factors Affecting B-12 Deficiency. 68
Dietary Deficiency of Vitamin B-12 69
Malabsorption of B-12 70

Chapter Nine: Minerals **71**

Mineral Content of the Body 71
Uses in the Body. 71
Requirements 72
Pica 72
Specific Minerals 72
   Calcium. 72
   Sodium. 73
   Iron 74
   Iodine 76
   Selenium. 76
   Aluminum. 76
   Magnesium. 76
   Phosphorus. 76
   Zinc 76
   Trace Elements. 77

Chapter Ten: Condiments, Additives, and Herbs **79**

Stimulating and Sedating Foods 79
Spices 79
Monosodium Glutamate 80
Chromosome Breakage. 80
Other Effects 80
Vinegar. 81
Baking Soda. 81
Eating Between Meals 81
Other Food Additives. 81

Chapter Eleven: Controls of Thirst and Appetite **87**

Water Requirements and Thirst 87
Drink, Drink, Drink 87
When Shall I Drink Fluids?. 87
Controls of Hunger and Appetite 88

Chapter Twelve: Digestion **89**

Functions of the Digestive Tract 89
Mouth. 89
   Teeth 89
   Tongue 89
   The Salivary Glands 89
The Esophagus 89
Stomach. 90
Duodenum. 90
Small Intestine. 91
Colon or Large Intestine. 92
Liver and Gallbladder. 93
Major Functions of the Liver 93
Major Functions of the Pancreas. 93
General Principles of Digestion. 93
Fat Digestion and Absorption. 93
Protein Digestion and Absorption. 94
Psychological Factors Influencing Digestion. 94
Fecal Flora 95

Chapter Thirteen: Metabolism **97**

The Position of Enzymes in Metabolism 97
Basal Metabolism 97
Metabolism and Energy. 98

Chapter Fourteen: Endocrinology **99**

Adrenals. 99
Thyroid. 100
   Hyperthyroidism. 100
   Hypothyroidism. 100
   Cretinism 101
Menopause 101
   Foods Low in Estrogen-Like Sterols 102
   Osteoporosis 102

Chapter Fifteen: Diabetes, the Principal Disease of Metabolism

Accelerated Aging. 105
The Pima Indians 106
The Yemenite Jews. 106
The Eskimos and Diabetes 106
Juvenile Diabetes 108
The Hypoglycemic Syndrome Defined. 109
Treatment for Diabetes and the Hypoglycemic Syndrome. . . . 111
Foods Allowed. 112
Foods to Avoid 112
Questions Often Asked about the Hypoglycemic Syndrome. . . 113

Chapter Sixteen: Regular and Spare Diets **117**

The Weight of the Vegetarian 117
Function of Body Fat 117
Ideal Weight 117
Dangers of Overweight. 118
Help for the Overweight Person 118
Diets for Weight Reduction—Good and Bad. 119
Common Errors in Eating that Lead to Overweight 121
Summary of Thought Errors Leading to Overweight 122
Weight Control Routine 122
Main Dishes. 123
Eleven Aids to Prevent Overeating 123
Causes of Cravings. 124
Sample Menu for Reducing Diet 125
Underweight 125
Sprouting 125

Chapter Seventeen: Advice for Pregnant Vegetarians **127**

Diet. 127
Certain Alkaloids are Toxic 127
Alcohol and Other Drugs 128
Mental Attitude 128
Exercise 128
Clothing. 129

Chapter Eighteen: Vegetarian Diet in Childhood **131**

Generous Diet in Childhood 131
Breast Milk, Baby's First Food. 131
Nutrient Content of Human and Cow's Milk 132
Breastfeeding Good for Mother and Child 132
Specificity of the Milk of An Animal 132
Introducing Solid Foods. 133
Three Essential Food Groups 133
Weaning. 134
Don'ts for Feeding a Child 135

Appendix **137**

Index **151**

CHAPTER ONE

Why Be a Vegetarian?

Man Naturally a Vegetarian

Anatomy, physiology, and instinct all testify that man is by nature a fruit eating creature. Expressions from well-known naturalists voice the sentiment of most people who have made a careful study of the subject:

"The natural food of man, judging from his structure, consists of fruit, roots, and vegetables."—Cuvier

"No physiologist would dispute with those who maintain that man ought to live on a vegetarian diet." Dr. Spencer Thompson

"An excessive meat diet, while producing in life's first half extraordinary energy and restless activity, leaves the body a used up, empty shell after forty-five. It acts like a furnace with a forced draft." —Anonymous

"Simple fare and correctly prepared foods... will keep the human body the replica of the Divine form. It will not develop excessive fat or obnoxious pugnacity, but rather will it leave the mind free for the contemplation of life's highest ideals."[1]

Cosmetic Reasons for Being Vegetarian

Cosmetic purposes are, suprisingly, high on the list of reasons given for becoming a vegetarian. Aging of the skin and hair is less noticeable in vegetarians. The skin is more free from blemishes, the weight is lighter, the muscles and joints more supple. Many professional entertainers are vegetarians for this reason.

Religious Reasons

Many have experienced a clearer mind and a deeper spiritual life on a vegetarian diet. The lifestyle that often accompanies vegetarianism lends much support to this position. For this reason, many Easterners and those favoring a type of ascetic lifestyle adopt a vegetarian diet in order to cultivate the spiritual nature. Some, as in India, are vegetarians because of religious taboos. Members of the Vegan Society and others follow vegetarianism because of a benevolent spirit and concern over the cruelty and killing of animals in the commercial production of animal products.

Economic Reasons

Poverty is the compelling factor in the vegetarianism of a large part of the world's population—they simply cannot afford the extravagant food bill of those who use animal products. Beef protein costs more than soybean protein by a comparison factor of forty to one.[2]

Length of Life Before the Flood

All the nourishment found in the world today was made initially by plants. When one eats animal products, the nourishment received is secondhand. A high meat diet stimulates a rapid rate of growth, predisposing to a shorter lifespan.[3] Animal protein tends to run our engines at a high rate of speed, even when we are at rest, promoting accelerated aging. On man's original diet of fruit, nuts, legumes, and probably fruiting vegetables, the average recorded lifespan was 912 years.[4] Animal products were permitted in man's diet after the flood,[5] probably to shorten his lifespan and reduce his record of sinning, intemperance, fatigue, pain, sorrow, and fear. God did not want man to perfect a sophistication that hundreds of years in sin would produce. And hundreds of years were not necessary for him to indicate his choice for his eternal destiny and to perfect a righteous character.

The following figures show the average length of life was 912 years when man was on a vegetarian diet for the nine generations before the flood as recorded in Genesis 5:3-32 and 9:29. The average for the first ten generations after the flood, when animal products were used as food, was but 317 years.[6]

Nine Generations Before the Flood

Name	Age
Adam	930
Seth	912
Enos	905
Cainan	910
Mahalaleel	895
Jared	962
Enoch (Translated)	
Methuselah	969
Lamech	777
Noah	950
	8,210
Average	912 years

Ten Generations After the Flood

Name	Age
Shem	600
Arphaxad	438
Salah	433
Eber	464
Peleg	239
Reu	239
Serug	230
Nahor	148
Terah	205
Abraham	175
	3,171
Average	317 years

"And Haran died before his father Terah in the land of his nativity,..."[7] One would deduce from this scripture that until about the tenth generation after the flood, it was so unusual a thing for a child to die before his father that special mention is made of the fact in Holy Writ.

Length of life from Shem to Abraham, ten generations, declined from an average of 912 down to the 175 years of Abraham's life.[8] At the exodus from Egypt, 430 years later, it had fallen to about the present length of "threescore years and ten."[9] The father's age at which his first child was born was also greatly shortened—from 100 years for Shem, who was born before the flood, to around 30 to 35 in the first generations after the flood.

An Historically Reliable Diet

Most of mankind has used near-vegetarian diets for all of recorded human history except for the past few centuries. We can conclude that the most successful dietary ever tried by man is the vegetarian diet. Most of the strong conquerors of the natural resources of this world developed their hardiness on a diet principally of fruits, vegetables and whole grains. The Creator designed man to be vegetarian, the original diet for man being given in Genesis 1:29. God has instructed man to subdue and have dominion over the earth and its vast resources.[10] Modern man, with his very rich diet, is progressively entering into degenerative disease and loss of ambition, as well as emotional instability all of which make him more susceptible to neurotic behavior, war, crime, and family upheaval.

Health Reasons

In America, the principal motivating factor in adopting vegetarian diets appears to be health. Seventh-day Adventists, university students, health enthusiasts, and endurance athletes fall in this category. The Chinese coolie, although not large of stature, will draw a load of freight at the speed of a horse's trot for a distance of from 30 to 40 miles at a time. His diet consists of rice, dates, vegetables, and rarely a small portion of fish. The Hindu messengers, who carry dispatches long distances day after day, live principally on rice. The Irish peasant, who ranks among the most active of men, subsists chiefly on potatoes, buttermilk, and simply cooked vegetables. The native Andean Indian, after carrying on his shoulders burdens of 200 pounds, is able to do a day's work of far greater magnitude than most of our ordinary laborers. His food is largely bananas and whole meal cereal!

The blood chemistries are more likely to be in the ideal range with a vegetarian diet. A great deal of publicity has been given to the low blood cholesteral levels, low uric acid levels, and good kidney and liver function of vegetarians. Not a small item in the eyes of most Americans is that weight levels of vegetarians are usually well below that of non-vegetarians. Hemoglobin levels in the blood are rarely elevated above normal, a common finding in non-vegetarians.

Perhaps part or all of the various reasons given

above are pushing many into vegetarianism. As food prices soar and as animal diseases transmissible to man increase, thinking people everywhere are becoming vegetarians. Hardly a week goes by that some new person is not heard to say: "I have decided to become a vegetarian. What should I do to get a balanced diet?"

Vegetarianism Discussed: Nutritional Superiority

A report of the Select Committee on Nutrition and Human Needs of the United States Senate reported that "our diets have changed radically within the last 50 years, with very great and often harmful effects on health. These dietary changes represent as great a threat to public health as smoking. Too much fat, too much sugar or salt...are linked directly to heart disease, cancer, obesity, and stroke, among other killer diseases....Six of the ten leading causes of death in the United States have been linked to our diet....In the early 1900's, almost 40 percent of our caloric intake came from fruit, vegetables, and grain(s)....Today...a little more than 20 percent of calories come from these sources."[11]

It is obvious that major reforms are needed if we are to avoid slipping further into the dangerous epidemic of degenerative disease. Generally, vegetarians are making decided steps in diet reform. Usually a vegetarian is a well-informed person, with much more knowledge than his physician on the subject of nutrition. Most physicians cannot give counsel to their vegetarian patients in this area. Therefore, the special needs of the vegetarian must be met from some other source. Care must be taken to use common sense with diet, as errors are costly both to pocketbook and to health. It seems proper to look at large population groups or past generations of vegetarians, and then to feel confident in the experiences that have promoted health in our forebears for centuries.

Authorities in nutrition differ substantially regarding their evaluation of the adequacy of a vegetarian diet, depending on their vested interests. If one reads the publications of the United Fresh Fruit and Vegetable Association, it can be easily understood that the vegetarian diet is more than adequate, and people in the United States are certainly eating too much animal protein.[12] The National Poultry and Meat Association and the Dairy Council, however, are unlikely to make such admissions. Biased opinions in others are often a result of successful propaganda by such vested in-

terest groups. These groups are among the most influential in the world, and can sway attitudes and opinions by their excellent educational efforts. They happily furnish their beautifully designed charts and visual aids that impart an attitude of authority to college nutrition instructors, county health departments, textbook writers, and health educators anywhere.

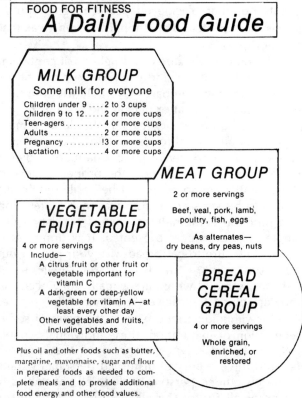

Sample of a chart similar to those which can be freely obtained in large, impressive, 4-color cards, vividly illustrated, but overemphasizing animal products to the point of promoting the epidemic of degenerative diseases we are now experiencing. The American Heart Association recommends for all Americans no more than 5 servings of meat per week. Yet this National Dairy Council chart urges "2 or more servings" daily.
See beautiful color chart page 14, Bogert & Briggs, 9th ed., Saunders

Actually, most nutritionists are beginning to recognize the nutritional superiority of certain vegetarian diets. The greatest battle lines, at present, are drawn over the vegan diet. Protein is a principal weapon used to attack vegetarian diets; but it should be recognized that the protein requirement of a 150-pound man may be satisfied with the daily ingestion of only approximately 30 grams of protein (one tablespoon holds about 15 grams), or the protein in about four slices of whole wheat bread.[13] A vegetarian woman with a modest food intake will probably get 40 to 50 grams, and hefty men around 50 to 150! Even dogs, with their high metabolism, don't need much protein. In *Time* magazine, Barbara Woodhouse, the famous dog trainer in England, said modern dogs eat too much protein. Dog food is advertised at 20-27% protein, which Ms. Woodhouse says makes dogs hyperactive and schizophrenic. She says they need no more than 14% protein.[14]

The United States Department of Agriculture points out that black-eyed peas can give you 7.2 grams more protein than chopped sirloin steak (half cup portions).[15]

The biological value of a single meal containing a combination of rice and beans or corn and beans, as the main dish, compares favorably with the same meal containing meat or milk as the main dish.

To allay unnecessary fears, it should be remembered that all natural foods contain all the essential amino acids in greater or lesser quantities.[16] By eating a wide variety of foods, the proper balance of the essential amino acids will be easily obtained.[17] It should be stressed that all reasonable diets contain foods in combinations. Menus consisting of a single food are never presented. It is unnecessary to say, "Be sure to eat bread with your peanut butter." While there are bizarre individuals in all cultures, some of whom are actually convinced that they are doing themselves and their children a service by withholding food even to the point of severe retardation of maturation, these individuals should not be classed as vegetarians, since they properly fall into the category of disturbed personality traits. Some misguided persons exclude all vegetables or grains or all fruits. The all raw diet is difficult for most people to digest, and many children will starve or nearly starve while consuming an all raw diet. We treated a nice lady in her sixties who developed pellagra after twelve years on an all raw diet. Despite vigorous attempts to bring her out of the pellagra and its associated mental illness, we were able only partially to reverse her condition. She was eventually admitted to a mental hospital by her family where she died a few weeks later. We felt she had permanently damaged her digestive tract and nervous system by the prolonged use of a restricted variety of raw foods.

Commenting on an article in the *Journal* of the *American Medical Association,*[18] Dr. Glen Toppenberg states: "The majority of populations in economically less-developed countries of Asia, Africa, and Latin America habitually subsist on inexpensive vegetarian diets, made up of high starch and grains. This may well make up the greater proportion of our world's population. To illustrate

vegetarian child-raising firsthand, my three children are now the third generation of my family to have never tasted meat, and it certainly has not been detrimental to our health." Yet, occasionally a child will have failure to thrive while on a vegetarian diet. When a child, whose parents eat a diet dangerously high in fats, animal products, and sweets develops failure to thrive, an educational program is developed for the parents. But when the vegan parents face the same feeding problem nutritionists sometimes suggest employing the statutes of child abuse, if the parents do not change their food tradition. Through the years it has seemed better to us to treat both groups of parents alike and have an educational program for both groups, teaching parents of children having feeding problems and failure to thrive how to feed their particular child. These problems are not unique to vegetarians; in fact, they are less often encountered.

Those who use a vegan diet, no animal products, can feel confident that they have a balanced and adequate diet only if they use common sense in its application. As with all other parents, vegan parents will sometimes become baffled by their child and a feeding problem will ensue. Of course, to deny a child good quality food which has been requested, or to fail to provide a sufficient quantity of food for a growing child when it is available is unthinkable. However, in the overwhelming majority of cases, it is sympathetic guidance and correction of misconceptions that is needed rather than litigation.

If parents are psychotic and fail to give their children adequate nourishment, whatever the weight of the child and whatever the diet tradition used, measures should be taken one way or the other to protect the child. If milk, pork and doughnuts are the sole diet of a fat, malnourished child, the body weight of the child and the expensiveness of the food should not lead educational services astray in dealing with the situation. I well remember the case of a 10-year-old boy who came to autopsy in our department of pathology who had terminal cirrhosis of the liver from drinking alcoholic drinks. His parents had thought he was "so cute" when drunk. This practice had gone on since the child was two. Proper dealing with the parents early in the course of this boy's life would have avoided such a tragic outcome of the parents' perverted ideas.

It is our belief that most vegan parents are far better educated on nutrition and more concerned than the average parents, and could, in most cases, be successfully educated to a proper dietary for their children. Certainly, to even threaten to take children away from their parents or threaten to bring child abuse charges against conscientious parents who are struggling to do what they believe to be right, is in itself an irresponsible and ethically incorrect use of authority. Far better to start with education!

There are certain cautions strict vegetarians should observe, such as that of getting adequate calories. In the strict vegetarian, these calories will be derived from unrefined grains, legumes, nuts, seeds, a variety of vegetables including the leafy kind, and an abundance of fruits. If the diet is unbalanced with too much refined starchy food and too many cereals, or if the caloric intake is insufficient to maintain fuel requirements, the strict vegetarian may run into trouble.[19]

There has been a general departure from well-known and thoroughly tried food patterns accepted for centuries. These departures carry some dangers for modern societies, dangers that are easily defined and readily avoided. Examples of these departures lie in the areas of too much fat (margarine, mayonnaise, and cooking fats), too much sugar, and the use of artificial coloring and flavoring agents. Convenience foods and junk foods are typical of these recent introductions into the food marketing practices that injure health. Most of these dangers are not risks for the vast majority of vegetarians, as an exposure to the danger is never a consideration in their lifestyle. Special dangers which might more naturally involve vegetarians are such as the use of uncooked, coarse vegetables like kale (which contains thiaminase, causing the breakdown of thiamin). Disorders from these greens have not been described in humans, but a nervous system disease called "star-gazing" in ruminant animals as a result of degeneration of the brain (cerebro-cortical necrosis) has been reported when the animals eat large quantities of forage crops containing antinutritional factors such as thiaminase.

Food properly selected, stored, and prepared will provide all the nutrients necessary for good nutrition. The RDA (recommended daily allowance) is set by the Committee on Dietary Allowances of the Food and Nutrition Board, after estimating the needs of all Americans. The RDA is changed frequently, sometimes radically, as estimates of nutrient needs change through the years. We should not oppose investigation and clarification. On the other hand, when estimates of nutrient requirements are

a great departure from historically recognized requirements, or are outside the realm of reason, one should simply do what is reasonable and keep an open mind.

Not only are plant proteins adequate, but they actually have several advantages. These advantages include an associated lower quantity and better quality of fat and a higher quantity of fiber complexed with the protein and fat. Of the twenty amino acids from which proteins are built, eight must be supplied to man by the leaves of green plants. After production through energy gained by photosynthesis by the leaves of green plants, these amino acids are then stored in seeds, tubers, and other parts of the plant and may be taken up by the animals to be stored in their flesh or organs. Only 8-20% of the protein from plant sources fed to farm animals can be recovered as protein for human nutrition.[20] It is unlikely that protein deficiency will develop in apparently healthy adults on a diet in which cereals and vegetables supply adequate calories.[21]

The Tarahumara Indians live in the High Sierra mountains of Chihuahua in Mexico, about 300 miles from El Paso, Texas. They are among the finest endurance runners in the world, if not the ultimate in this regard. They sometimes engage in a marathon race of 100 to 200 miles, all done in rough mountainous terrain, while kicking a lightweight wooden ball, often in the dark. Friends carry torches so the runner can see the ball. Formerly, Tarahumaras caught deer by chasing them on foot until *the deer* dropped from exhaustion. Yet, some nutritionists in the United States would say that they are on a mere starvation diet. They rarely, if ever have meat, milk, eggs, or fruit. Their total caloric intake is about 2250 to 2800 calories daily, consisting mainly of beans, corn, and vegetables. It is abundantly adequate in protein, yet protein comprises only 13-14% of their caloric intake, with 96% of the protein coming from plant sources. Despite this, these men develop the most remarkable physical stamina known to humans.

From the experience of the Tarahumaras, we can say that a high animal protein diet is definitely not needed and is possibly even a detriment to proper development of athletic stamina. The men are short, slightly over five feet, and none over 5'9", weighing between 104 and 163 pounds. They have only about 7% body fat, and a maximum would probably be less than 12%.[22]

Aging Process Slower in Vegetarians

Osteoporosis is the bane of life for many post-menopausal women. Vegetarian women, however, suffer far less than do others from this disabling disorder. At approximately age 69, vegetarians appear to suffer no further decline in bone density. In contrast, those who eat a mixed diet have a bone density which continues to decline.[23]

Antioxidants, such as selenium, vitamin C, and vitamin E reduce the aging effects of diet and various traumatic events of life. Antioxidants are found more abundantly in foods of a vegetarian type than in animal products.[24]

Some Physiological Effects of Meat Eating

Because of meat ammonia, intestinal cancer can be expected to be of a higher incidence in persons who eat meat. Ammonia is one of the natural waste products of protein digestion; the more protein eaten the more ammonia produced. Ammonia has been recognized as harmful to man and animals. It increases virus infection, and, of course, some viruses are known to cause cancer. Ammonia slows the growth of normal cells more than that of cancer cells. Ammonia changes the character of ribonucleic acid as well as the rate that the nucleic acid thymidine can be utilized to synthesize deoxyribonucleic acid, an important complex molecule of all nuclei. Cell turnover is increased by ammonia. The higher the cell turnover, the greater the chance that the cell will become cancerous.

The constant exposure to ammonia over the course of a lifetime probably causes serious damage. Intestinal cancer tends to increase as the amount of ammonia production increases.[25] There are some food supplements that increase the amount of ammonia formed: protein supplements, soy isolates, food yeasts, etc. Ammonia is also formed in the urine when urine is retained for too long a period of time in the bladder. A good health habit is to keep the bladder emptied, and also reduce the concentration of urine by drinking water freely, so that the cleansing of the bladder can reduce the exposure to ammonia.

Chemicals which cause mutations in the chromosomes of cells (mutagens) are generally more likely to cause cancer. Tests were performed to determine if vegetarians are less likely to have mutagens in their feces. It was found that vegetarians have significantly lower levels of fecal mutagens than non-vegetarians. Urban, white South Africans, a population at high risk for colon cancer, have a rate of mutagens in their fecal samples of 19%, whereas only 2% of urban blacks and none of the rural blacks showed mutagens. Both of the lat-

ter are low risk groups for colon cancer.[26]

Diseases from meat include trichinosis, cysticercosis, salmonellosis, etc. Seafood can cause serious illness such as hepatitis A, typhoid, cholera, vibriosis, paralytic and neurotoxic shellfish poisoning, and gastrointestinal illness of unknown cause.[27] Hand infections occur in butchers from contact with meat.[28]

Individuals on a vegetarian diet are generally healthy if they eat appropriately varied diets. As a rule, they continue to be employed at their jobs about ten to twenty years later in life than non-vegetarians, depending on the occupation. In physical testing, the endurance of vegetarians is greater than that of meat-eating individuals.[29] Nutritional deficiencies, particularly in vegetarian children, can easily be prevented by very basic and rudimentary knowledge. Those who question the overuse of animal products, processed and refined foods, white flour, white sugar and food additives may demonstrate their reverence for human life on this planet by recognizing current nutrition research[30] which emphasizes the advantage of the vegetarian diet.

One study showed that rats fed a strictly vegetarian diet reproduced and lived as long as others, even when continued on the diet for several generations, although they were smaller in size.[31] In humans, the fecal excretion of fats and bile acids, as well as the presence in the stomach and intestine of various bacteria, change for the better when a person switches from a meat-based to a vegetarian diet.[32]

The way the body handles drugs and other foreign chemicals is influenced by what one eats. In the liver some metabolic transformations occur at a slower rate in vegetarians. The liver apparently functions in a different gear for vegetarians. According to a study done on vegetarian immigrants to the United Kingdom from the Indian subcontinent[33] vegetarians metabolize certain drugs more slowly than do non-vegetarians. This fact may explain why vegetarians rarely become drug addicts, use alcohol, or smoke. Vegetarians should warn their physicians and anesthesiologists that they will not need as much of a drug or anesthesia as is generally needed for others. Many vegetarians report that they are drugged for days longer than others after routine anesthetic experiences.

Protective Value of a Simple Diet

Persons who eat a high fiber, vegetarian diet tend to excrete fat at higher levels indicating that fat is being bound by the fiber and carried out of the body. Therefore, less fat is absorbed from the food. This may explain the low body weight of many vegetarians,[34, 35] as well as their low blood fats. Unsaturated fats of grains and legumes protect against foreign chemicals, as do vitamins C and A, zinc, magnesium, copper, and calcium.

There are no purines in fats, but fats may be very difficult for patients suffering with gout to handle. Apparently fat interferes with the normal routes of excretion of uric acid. Alcohol behaves in the same way that fat does in preventing excretion of uric acid. Overweight is an invitation to a high uric acid. Most animal proteins cause the uric acid to go up. Yeast, both bakers and brewers, contains a high concentration of purines, inviting a high uric acid. In summary, we can say that a diet high in animal products, fat, alcohol, excessive calories, and yeast products can lead to gout. Since gout is a disorder precipitated by excessive blood levels of uric acid it would seem that one method to help the situation would be to reduce the intake of foods high in purines, and secondly to increase methods of uric acid excretion, especially in individuals who may have tendencies toward gout. Therefore the obvious thing to do to treat or prevent gout is to avoid high purine foods--all meat, poultry and fish as well as the other situations that invite a high uric acid. Members of the vegetable kingdom that have a slightly increased likelihood of causing the uric acid to go up are the legume family (beans, lentils, peas, and peanuts), as well as mushrooms, spinach, and asparagus.

There is no danger of protein deficiency even after eliminating the foods mentioned. Wheat, corn, rice, all other grains, the many products made from grains such as pastas (spaghetti, macaroni, and noodles), bulgar, and a large variety of fruits and vegetables contain sufficient proteins to supply all of one's needs. Dr. Marian Nestle, associate dean at the University of California School of Medicine in San Francisco told a group of family physicians at their 33rd Annual Convention that a "wide variety of unprocessed high-carbohydrate foods" is the diet recommended for "normal and therapeutic diets". This diet, she said, includes "fruits, vegetables, whole grain cereals that are relatively low in calories, fat, sugar, salt, and food additives, and contains relatively high amounts of vitamin, minerals, and fiber."[36] Drinking plenty of water and eating freely of fruits will help rid the body of excess uric acid. A fast is not recommended when the uric acid is already very high, or one is

in a gouty attack, as the rapid weight loss can temporarily increase the uric acid in the blood. Strawberries and cherries are reported to make the uric acid go down, and should be used generously in the diet of those whose uric acid is elevated. Flowers of the broom plant from which a tea is made can help gout.

Another protective effect of a vegetarian diet is found in the fact that Brussels sprouts or cabbage stimulate the intestinal metabolism of phenacetin, a pain-killing drug.[37] Therefore to rid the body of phenacetin more quickly than is normally done by the liver, foods of the cabbage family should be eaten.

A diet high in fruits and vegetables appears to protect against the production of kidney stones.[38] Eating excessively of meat is believed to be a major cause of renal stones.[39]

The reports of other physicians confirm our observations that white blood cell counts are lower in vegetarians than in others, and are generally between 3500 and 5000 as a normal range. It should be pointed out that individuals who exercise briskly and who have a generally high level of good health usually have low white blood cell counts.

A study of 4,264 men showed that the number of white blood cells customarily found in the blood is higher in smokers, more notably in those who inhale. There is an increase of about 30% in the leukocyte count for heavy smokers who inhale as compared to nonsmokers. The increase is in granulocytes, lymphocytes, and monocytes.[40]

The number of white blood cells circulating at any one time should be low, just as the pulse rate ideally should be low. Such activities as exercise increase the pulse (*and* the white blood cell count) during exercising. However, as a result of having exercised, when physically trained people are in the resting state, the pulse rate is low, causing a reduction in the work load of the heart. *Low resting levels* of white blood cells similarly *reduce the demands* made on the bone marrow to produce many new cells.

Meat eating alters blood chemistries. The impurities from the metabolism of the animal itself, the pollutants from the environment, the hormones of fear produced by transport and slaughter, the toxins and drugs to which the animal has been exposed --all these enter the bloodstream of the person who eats the flesh of the animal. One study showed that the serum creatinine levels were elevated in healthy volunteers fed cooked meat.[41]

Creatinine is a waste product excreted by the kidneys; the increased level puts a greater tax on the kidneys.

Many people began to turn to the vegetarian diet in response to concern over the poisoning by PBB'S (polybrominated biphenyls) in 1973 to 1976. The outbreak occurred in Michigan due to the accidental substitution of a toxic fire retardant (Firemaster) for a feed supplement (Nutrimaster), resulting in contamination of milk, eggs, poultry, and beef. At least 8,000 Michigan residents are known to have been exposed.[42]

Leukemia Incidence Higher in Cattle Country

Vegetarians generally have less cancer of all kinds than those who use animal products. Iowa, noted for its beef and dairy industries, has an incidence of leukemia higher than that of the general population. Dr. Kelley J. Donham, a veterinarian from the Institute of Agricultural Medicine of the University of Iowa, has found that more cases of acute lymphocytic leukemia, the most common type of leukemia in children, occurs in the most rural parts of the state where dairy cattle are most numerous. Further, the leukemia in the humans parallels lymphosarcoma (a cancerous condition) in cattle. A virus that can be transmitted from cow to cow and cow to humans is the cause of the disease. In those counties having the most cases of lymphosarcoma in the cattle there is about 70% excess of acute lymphocytic leukemia in the human population. Humans are exposed to the disease through meat, milk, cheese, eggs, and direct contact with animals.[43] Another way that a vegetarian diet is superior to a diet containing animal products is that the vegetarian diet does not expose humans to the serious disabling or death dealing infectious diseases of animals.

Breast and Bowel Cancer Less in Vegetarians

Breast cancer is 28% less for vegetarians in California than for other adult females in the same area. Reduced risk of bowel cancer is seen in vegetarians, possibly because of conversion of cholic acid in the enterophepatic cycle,[44] or because fiber attaches toxic substances that act as cancer producing agents, or because the refuse is carried more quickly from the bowel in vegetarians, resulting in briefer exposure of toxic substances in contact with the bowel. A number of bile acids have been shown to be carcinogenic. Fats, bile acids, and the fecal bacteria are higher in people on a mixed diet than

those on a strict vegetarian diet.[45] Children thrive on a vegetarian diet, and it is compatable with above average mental development.[46]

Vegetarian women excrete 2-3 times more estrogens in feces than do those who use animal products, and at any given time non-vegetarian women can be expected to have a blood level of certain fractions of estrogens 50% higher than vegetarian women. The same low levels can be observed in fractions of estrogens found in the urine of vegetarians as compared to non-vegetarians. These low levels of estrogens probably explain part of the lower incidence of breast cancer in vegetarian women.[47]

No Diabetes and Plenty of Good Teeth

A major advantage of the strict vegetarian diet is the virtual absence of diabetes. Diabetes is highly uncommon among vegans, probably partly because they are rarely fat. In the train of this advantage comes a number of blessings, not the least of which is good teeth. If you count the teeth before the age of 30, the average non-diabetic will have 27 teeth and the average diabetic 24. During the decade after the age of 30, the average non-diabetic has lost only three more teeth, while the average diabetic has lost ten more. The factors that are detrimental to dental health are known also to be serious ones in the mental illness profile as well. They are also known to be detrimental to the cardiovascular system. People who eat foods high in niacin, such as those on a vegetarian diet, tend to have fewer psychological complaints [48] and fewer heart attacks.

How to Feed a Hungry World

Not the least in the considerations of a diet for a hungry world is the economy of the vegetarian diet. Over one billion people are hungry all the time, and that number is expected to triple in the next ten years. [49] Since it costs about ten times as much to support a person on a meat-based diet as on a vegetarian diet, all individuals should be encouraged to grow as much as possible of their own food and learn to subsist on a vegetarian diet. By far the greatest proportion of the massive grain production in North America goes to feed animals, not humans. As our precious fuel supplies continue to dwindle, this fact will take on ever-increasing significance.

All livestock, pets, small caged animals, and even aquarium fish are increasingly competitive with humans for food in a hungry world with mounting difficulties in finding enough food. The food consumed by household pets in Britain alone would feed 700,000 starving persons, by 1974 estimates. About half of United States households contains a pet. The dog/cat ratio is about 5:3. Cats eat less than dogs and are more able to forage for food such as mice, reptiles, birds, dead animals, refuse, and waste food. [50]

We need ways to cut the cost of living in our overpopulated world. The vegetarian diet accomplishes this feat by reducing both food and illness costs. The bill for being sick goes up every year. In 1929, 3.5 billion dollars were spent for all medical care. At that time, such a large expenditure was felt to be a great drain on the resources of the people, about 10 cents per person per day. However, in 1968 the cost was 68 cents! Three short years later in 1971, medical care costs in the United States were nearly 30 billion dollars more than in 1968. That's 79 billion dollars![48] With such a meteoric rise in cost, there are those who might expect an astronomical improvement in national health; but actually, on investigation we found the reverse to be true. The general level of health dwindled; more people were in hospitals, nursing homes, and intermediate care units than ever before. In the book "How You Can Live Six Extra Years," Lewis Walton says "Soon, unless some miracle occurs, the whole system will collapse. Medical care as we have come to expect it will simply be unavailable at any price."[51] Sweeping changes are needed in lifestyle, in diet, and in our understanding of economy if we are to survive.

How People Become Vegetarians

Unless one who aspires to become a vegetarian is a member of a group having several generations of established vegetarians, the person usually evolves along the path of becoming a vegetarian by first dropping meat, then fish and eggs, and later milk. The individuals who have passed through successive generations of vegetarians usually do not have any nutritional problems along their vegetarian pathway; whereas, the so-called "new-vegetarians" may occasionally experience some problems.

A study of 100 new vegetarians revealed that 35% had become vegetarians for health reasons (alertness, mental function, and general good health, as well as long-term prevention of cancer, stroke, and heart disease). Ethical reasons were stated in 25%, metaphysical reasons in 14%, ecological reasons in 8%, and unstated in 18%.[52]

CHAPTER TWO

Nutrition, Longevity, and Usefulness

Productivity, the Objective of Nutrition

"Let it ever be kept before the mind that the great object of hygenic reform is to secure the highest possible development of mind and soul and body."[53] The levels of function of the human body vary all the way from the point of the greatest possible satisfaction to the individual and the finest ability to be productive and creative in his society to the point of feebleness and death. Between these two extremes lie many intermediate points. It is a rare individual who realizes his fullest ability to grow and develop his maximum capacity in mental productivity, his deepest growth along spiritual lines, and who experiences perfect freedom from disease and other discomforts throughout his lifetime.

It is of interest that most schools of home economics in the United States have departments of nutrition while most medical schools, at least until very recently, do not. While physicians have long been looked on as the guardians of public health, nutritional science, that most basic of all physiological sciences, has been neglected by medical practitioners. At least 30% of the population of the United States shows some evidence of malnutrition, sometimes undernutrition, but most commonly selected overnutrition. One of the great aims of nutrition is to prolong the vitality of the prime of life into the later years. The major advantage youth has over old age is health and strength. Old age carries the advantage in all other ways. Experience, social development, character development, and spiritual understanding increase with age and should make life constantly more satisfying and productive. Unfortunately, many disorders and diseases develop with age and cause life to be unproductive and blighted as the thoughts become entirely occupied with various discomforts. "There are men and women of excellent natural ability who do not accomplish half of what they might if they would exercise self-control in the denial of appetite."[54]

The Basic Food Groups: Historical Considerations

Today, because of sophisticated processing and storage techniques, it is possible to travel from coast to coast at any season of the year with hardly a change in eating habits, despite changes in regional and seasonal food production. It has not always been so. Most early immigrants from Europe were accustomed to a limited, monotonous diet even in the summer. In the winter, diets often became a round of never-changing meals such as bread and greens at one meal and beans and corn at the next. Meat was an infrequent main dish, occurring usually less than twice weekly. Only a handful of vegetables were known in Europe prior to the 16th century. These included beets, carrots, radishes, turnips, and parsnips, plus cabbages, onions, leeks, and lentils. Fruits and berries were available only during a short harvest period. The standard grains were wheat, barley, oats, and rye.

Breakfast in America was early and light, consisting of bread, hominy grits, and fruit in season. Thinly sliced roast and ham would be served occasionally in more elegant homes. The mid-day dinner was the big meal of the day and contained ham, greens, pumpkin, and potatoes. Milk was scarce, as cows "dried up." Supper was bread and butter and some fruit, if available. Sweet potatoes and cabbages were major items. The cook was tied to the calendar and clock.

In America, on southern plantations, the common people ate sweet potato, black-eyed peas, collard greens, salted fish in winter, and sometimes fresh beef. In some sections of the South, fresh corn, corn syrup, corn bread, hoecake, grits, and Indian pudding made from corn meal were staples along with cucumber pickles, cabbage, and meats.

There have been many methods used by nutritionists in different countries to attempt to make the matter of meal planning easier. These methods have usually emphasized the grouping of foods and the recommendation of those that should be taken daily in the dietary in order to avoid deficiencies of nutrients. In the United States, through the years, the number of food groups considered essential for daily consumption has dwindled until now the nutritionist usually teaches that there are four basic groups promoted as essential: milk, meat, vegetable-fruit, and bread-cereal. In the not too distant past, we had the basic seven, and then the basic five generally taught as daily essentials for well-nourished persons.

The groupings have always encouraged over-consumption of more concentrated foods and have neglected the fruits and vegetables of which we are told "ye may freely eat." As knowledge of nutrition has increased, dependence on animal products has diminished. Because animals have become progressively more diseased, and the entire spread of nutrients available in the four groups has become more universally available, many concerned persons, among them certain Seventh-day Adventist nutritionists, have taught for over 100 years that no more than three food groups are essential for nutrition. One Adventist health educator said around 1900 that "...it is high time that we were educating ourselves to subsist upon fruits, grains, and vegetables."[55] When one's work is chiefly mental or if heavy pressures weigh one down, to eat only fruits and grains for a few days will be beneficial . "Fruits, used with thoroughly cooked bread two or three days old, which is more healthful than fresh bread, slowly and thoroughly masticated, will furnish all that the system requires."[56] When brain work is especially heavy or one is worried, a fruit diet, alone, for several days will be beneficial. All elements required to build good blood are found in these three food groups. "The simple grains, fruits of the trees, (and) vegetables, have all the nutritive properties necessary to make good blood."[57] It is a fact that many large families of animals and tremendous human population groups live from birth to death on these three food groups with only minute quantities, if any, of such other food types as nuts or animal products (meat, milk, eggs, and cheese.)

Essential Foods

There is no such thing as an essential food. There are essential nutrients. We may reject a certain food, but its essential nutrients can be obtained from another food. Example: Milk is a food containing essential nutrients. One may substitute foods such as greens, whole grains, legumes, and

root vegetables in order to obtain the same essential nutrients. There was a time when the nutrients in milk were not known, and proper substitutes could not be supplied. At that time. Seventh-day Adventists taught: "The time has not come to say that the use of milk and eggs should be wholly discarded. There are poor families whose diet consists largely of bread and milk. They have little fruit, and cannot afford to purchase the nut foods. In teaching health reform...we are to meet the people where they are. Until we can teach them how to prepare health...foods that are palatable, nourishing, and yet inexpensive, we are not at liberty to present the most advanced propositions regarding health reform diet."[58]

From 1910 to 1930 that picture changed and even reversed. Now the less expensive vegetables, whole grains, and fruits are readily accessible even to the poor. It is easy to teach anyone to prepare balanced meals from these three food groups, thus placing the people in an advanced position, ahead of the food shortages already developing. We now know enough to make a balanced dietary from the three groups that do not include animal products. During the same period mentioned above, changes occurred in the social and economic structure to enable us to present the most advanced position in healthful dietary. Transportation has so improved that fresh vegetables can be obtained the year around, even within the arctic circle. The monotony of the winter diet has been relieved, and virtually the same menu can be served in January as in July.

Another change that has altered the former picture is that the poor do not now have a yard with chickens or a cow roaming on open range. Milk and eggs are no longer the special foods of the poor, but are among the most expensive items in the dietary. The counsel to learn to subsist on fruit, vegetables, and whole grains more properly applies today.

Primary Rule of Nutrition

In any one food group there are different proportions of certain essential nutrients in the different foods of that group. A small amount of riboflavin but a large amount of calcium may be present in one food. The reverse is true in another food. However, by eating both foods, stores of both riboflavin and calcium may be built up. Therefore, the primary rule of nutrition is a wide variety of foods in as unrefined state as possible.

Having been made in the image and likeness of God, the human being is capable of thoughts of the same nature as his Creator. His physical being looks and functions like that of God. His moral nature can think and perceive after the fashion of his Creator. So that this moral nature will not be hindered in any way, God made the functioning of the body a matter that requires as little attention as possible. Eating should not consume the major part of the thoughts. In keeping with this objective, the Creator also provided for our food needs in such a way that by using common sense and an unperverted appetite, man could properly satisfy his nutritional needs from the vegetable kingdom.[59] We believe it is impossible on any reasonable, varied diet of fruits, vegetables, whole grains, and a few seeds or nuts to become undernourished, provided sufficient calories are taken to provide for energy needs.

Deterioration of the Earth at the Present

The earth shows evidence of leaching elements from its crust, interference with plant nutrients by toxic pollutants, atmospheric changes that may hinder utilization of nutrients and proper development of living forms, and other degenerative changes. The flora and fauna of this earth are greatly dwarfed in comparison to the original plants and animals of the earth. The first men who inhabited the earth were much taller and heavier than present men.[60] Women were proportionate but slightly smaller in stature than men. The flora of the earth was similarly proportioned in size by present standards. We have examples of fossilized ferns that reach ten to fifteen feet in height. Modern examples of the same species are only three to five feet. The immense stores of fossil fuels in the earth--coal, oil, gas--attest to the staggering quantities of plant life on earth before the flood. The present degenerative status of the earth is insufficient to maintain the growth of such giant sizes in either flora or fauna.

When individuals reach the size of giants today, it is a result of imbalanced physiological functions. Those who grow bigger, have the greatest muscular development, and the earliest sexual maturity generally have the onset of degenerative disease much earlier in life than those who eventually reach full maturity, but do not reach maximum physical development as early. Examples of this are the greater incidence of breast cancer in tall, overweight women than in short, thin women; and the earlier occurrence of coronary heart disease in men who matured rapidly into husky adults.

The length of time from birth to the age of reproduction can be called the "generation age." In 1880, the human generation age was 16.2 years. Each decade since then, we have reduced the generation age by six months to the present generation age of 11.7 years. Our high fat diet, with its large content of refined foods coupled with our generally practiced custom of force feeding children, offering snacks between meals, and urging children to eat three or four large meals daily have united to rush children into early, oversized maturity. Such practices encourage the onset of early senility. While three or four years may be gained at the beginning of life, eight to fifteen years may be lost at the end. This is to say nothing of the reduced productivity from battling various degenerative diseases from cavities to cardiac problems.

Dr. Lipset* in *Vogue*[61] for March, 1977, says: "Over-nutrition brings earlier menses; with it a hormone assault perhaps too prolonged for health. Laterlife weight gains also may threaten." In the same article it is stated: "Post-menopausal women produce estrogen in fatty tissue. Though the increase (in hormones) in the obese is small, its effects may be large enough to explain why they have more breast and endometrial cancer."

Dr. Ralph A. Nelson, Associate Professor of Nutrition at Mayo Medical School is reported in *Medical World News,* to say that excess protein in the diet produces no known benefit, can be injurious, and in all probability decreases the lifespan. Most people in this country eat twice as much protein as is needed. We need less than 0.8 grams per kilogram of body weight. Dr. Nelson suggests that the increased enzymatic activity and increased urea and albumin production that accompany increased protein intake represent idling our metabolic engines at a faster rate. In rats, the length of life appears to be inversely related to the amount of food consumed.[62] "The incidence of cancer of the large intestine among women of 23 countries is closely related to the per capita meat consumption."[63] There is an extremely impressive, positive correlation between dietary protein intake and cancer of the breast, colon, prostate, and pancreas. When protein intake is at or below the recommended daily allowance (RDA), the effect of many carcinogens such as aflatoxins is greatly decreased.[64]

The presence of too much linoleic acid, the principal fatty acid in such vegetable oils as corn oil and sunflower oil, acts as an initiator for cancer cells if the amount of total fats is also high. Therefore, both fat and protein can be said to increase the cancer risk. A good rule to follow is to take concentrated nutrients sparingly. Even vitamin C in

*Mortimer B. Lipset, director of The Clinical Center of The National Institute of Health.

high doses appears to be mutagenic (capable of altering the way cells reproduce).[65]

There are optimum quantities of food, optimum rates of growth, and optimum final statures. These optimum values are not synonymous with maximum values. Many Americans suffer severe and prolonged maladies that could have been prevented if from childhood they had taken a simpler and unrefined diet of fruits, vegetables, and whole grains.

Man Did Eat Angel's Food

Many major accomplishments of man have been started by those whose diets have been very plain, even austere. America was founded by men who struggled against the elements to establish small gardens under most unfavorable circumstances to supply a very limited variety of vegetables. Anciently, when the people of God were on the borders of the earthly Canaan, God led them into the wilderness where they could not get a flesh diet.[66] It was here that He gave them manna, "the bread of heaven." Manna was small and round like coriander seed, and could be prepared in such a way that it was pleasant to eat with either a fruit or a vegetable meal. On this simple diet, the people were less restless and rebellious than they would have been on a more stimulating diet. As food shortages and transportation problems place the world in great perplexity, we believe that the Lord intends to bring His people back to live on simple fruits, vegetables, and whole grains.

In this period of earth's history, more than any other time, people need clear heads and balanced emotions to face the momentous issues and their far-reaching consequences. Yet there was never a time when injurious food and drink have been so readily accessible and widely used. How serious our position, when judgments are made concerning our economy, ecology, or military matters by those whose perceptions are blunted by their diet and beverages!

John the Baptist, the representative of Elijah for his day, is a prototype of God's people in the end of time. John ate a strictly vegetarian diet, the pods from the locust tree and doubtless many native foods such as wild honey, berries, and tubers, as well as a variety of cultivated fruits, vegetables, and whole grains from the family gardens. It was predicted that a reform such as Elijah wrought would occur before the coming of the Messiah in the judgment.[67] That surely will include not only his strict morals, but also his simple diet.

These strong examples are given to the people of God in this last age of earth's history of their type of work and their lifestyle. These are found in the story of the children of Israel before entering Canaan, in Elijah with the widow of Zarephath [68,69,70] and John the Baptist,[71] all of whom were pure or nearly pure vegetarians before a major triumph. It seems reasonable to believe that the qualities needed in the world today--withstanding poverty, delay, and commercial boycott,[72] possessing patience, courage, endurance, and clearheadedness--could best be developed on a vegetarian diet and a simple lifestyle capable of producing vigorous men and women, even into advanced old age.

Human Appetite Hard to Control

It is true today, as in times past, that even God's people crave the "fleshpots of Egypt," and mourn and cry for the harmful foods popular in the world; although they know if they will bring their appetites under control God will take away all sickness from among them.[73] The degenerative "evil diseases of Egypt" would not be their lot, but would fall upon those who will not obey natural law.[74] However, because of the murmuring of the children of Israel immediately after they left Egypt and again just before they could have entered the earthly Canaan, they were not spiritually ready to go in and possess the Promised Land. They mourned and wept, murmured and complained, and were determined to have flesh food. So God allowed them to have the very diet He had in His mercy withheld from them. Quail were sent to them which they ate before it had been properly prepared--washed free of the blood—and the plague struck even while they were still chewing the flesh.

Their complaints stopped for a while. But even after they became accustomed to a simpler diet, they again demanded "the fleshpots of Egypt." The quail again flew into their camp. A large number of people died of the plague that followed the quail feast.[75]

It had not been God's intention that they should eat a stimulatory diet that would irritate the nerves and inflame the blood, making them unable to control their cravings and passions. It is interesting to ponder what role the quail feast played in the fear, frustration, and loss of ambition experienced a few days later when the spies returned from exploring the Promised Land. Of the twelve, only two were strong and brave enough to say: "We be well able to take it." All the others quaked in their boots and said: "There we saw the giants;"[76] and they could not be trusted to take over Canaan. At their demand God had sent the quail, "but sent leanness into their soul."[77] If we are determined to have hurtful foods to gratify appetite, God lets us have them, but we reap poverty of spirit.

Just as easily as God gave manna, He could have given them flesh, had it been essential for their health. But He who created, redeemed, and led them on the long wilderness journey to educate, discipline, and train them in correct habits, understood the influence of flesh eating upon the human system. He wanted to have a people who would, in their physical appearance, bear the Divine credentials, notwithstanding their long and difficult journey. The record attests to the fact that there was "not one feeble person" in all their tribes.[78] Imagine a modern city of one-and-a-half million or more with no hospitals, physicians, nurses, or physical therapy units! If we could duplicate their vegetarian diet and other features of their lifestyle, we might approach their stamina and health.

Meat is Stimulatory, Not Especially Strengthening

One of the great errors prevalent today is that muscular strength is dependent upon animal food. The simple whole grains, fruits, and vegetables have all the nutritive properties necessary to make good blood and strong muscle. Many nations have demonstrated this fact through the centuries to the present time. Not until the change in dietary habits that came with our present-day additives, colorings, manufactured flavorings, milling, refining, and concentrating, have there been difficulties in obtaining a simple diet.

We are composed of what we eat, and eating much flesh will actually diminish intellectual activity. Students could accomplish far more in their studies if they never ate meat. The animalistic nature of humans is strengthened by meat eating, and in just that proportion, the intellectual power is diminished. A religious life can be more successfully gained and maintained if the diet is vegetarian. The use of flesh meat stimulates more intensely the lustful propensities and thereby enfeebles the moral and spiritual nature. In this age of great unrest, criminality, and unleashed passions, we need to encourage and cultivate pure, chaste thoughts and to strengthen the moral powers rather that the lower nature and carnal powers. May God help us to awaken and set aside our self-indulgent appetites that we may live ennobled and enriched lives.

All kinds of inflammatory and cancerous or tumor-producing diseases are caused by meat eating. Yet since the harmful results of eating meat are delayed sometimes for several decades, the increased mortality caused by meat eating is not readily discerned. We have many good foods to satisfy hunger without turning to flesh foods to compose our bill of fare.

Eating Animal Products An Extravagance

Since there is so much poverty in the world, all concerned and benevolent people should study ways to eliminate expensive animal products from their menus and carefully use the money saved for the relief of hunger in depressed areas. We should bear in mind that when we eat animal products, we are but eating grains and vegetables secondhand. The animal receives from these foods the nutrition that makes it grow and readies it for market. The nutrients formerly in the grains and vegetable matter pass into the animal and become a part of its life. The thought of killing animals to be eaten is in itself revolting. If man's natural sense had not been perverted by the indulgence of appetite, human beings would not think of eating the flesh of animals.

With food prices soaring and more hungry people born daily into the world, it is easy to see that it is high time that we were educating ourselves to subsist upon fruits, whole grains, and vegetables. Those who understand nutrition and discern world conditions should go everywhere and train all who are willing to learn how to cook without using meat, milk, eggs, or cheese. We should use less and less animal products until they are not used at all. If we will begin discarding all unhealthful articles of diet, the taste will become educated in the right direction. We will develop a liking for fruits, grain, vegetables, and nuts. Our experience will soon revert to that designed for us in the beginning--the use of only the natural products from the earth.

Relish of Meals Surpasses Former Enjoyment

A more correct way of cooking can be learned by those who discard meat, and many healthful dishes can be prepared free from grease and animal products. A variety of simple dishes, perfectly healthful and nourishing, may be provided for the family aside from meat. When the taste is so educated, the person will discover that the enjoyment of food is far superior to that experienced when a more complicated and stimulating dietary was taken.

A proper quantity should be eaten; enough to sustain life and maintain strength. However, one need not eat so much as to burden the system or promote excessive weight. It is a mistake to believe that only a few stalks of celery and a few carrot curls will sustain life. Hearty men must have plenty of vegetables, fruits, and grains. Those who discard meat, after persevering for a few days, will find that they have greater powers of endurance than when they lived mostly on meat.

Several long distance runners have come to us for health counseling. Those who have tried a vegetarian menu invariably say they have a greater endurance on it than on a mixed dietary. The Chinese coolies and the Tarahumara Indians are famed for their unbelievable athletic feats, yet most of them subsist on a vegetarian diet. Many studies have revealed vegetarians to have superior endurance, some having over twice the endurance of non-vegetarians in the same geographic area and with the same ethnic background.

Never Call An Impoverished Diet Health Reform

Soft mushes, soups, porridge, and other foods containing a lot of water, but that do not have a generous caloric content, will not sustain life. When foods rich with animal products, grease, sugars, and refined proteins are removed from the dietary, one should not get the idea that he should live on soupy cereal and watered down stew. Those who work hard will be expending plenty of energy and must have a generous supply of food. A poverty-stricken diet, or one that shows evidence of unbalanced restrictions, should not be spoken of as a vegetarian diet but as an unfortunate diet of the poor, the ignorant, the careless, or the imbalanced.

Those who advocate health reform should never adopt an impoverished diet. To do so is not in harmony with the obvious intent of God in providing such an abundance of nourishing food. Good food makes good blood, but the adoption of an impoverished diet can cause disease which is difficult to cure, skeletal problems, deficiency diseases with degenerative changes, and mental aberrations. It is unfair for children to have parents who will not study this matter and supply for them a balanced diet of good quality food.

There are many ways for the diet to be improper. These may be complexity, nutrient deficiency and imbalances, concentration of nutrients or calories, an emphasis on animal products, extravagance, too much liquid food, meager calories, or rich and stimulating foods. Just because a diet is simple does not mean that it must be meager. On the other hand, simplicity does not give one license to overeat. The diet should be adapted to the climate in which a person lives, to the age of the person, to the occupation, to any physical diseases, and even to the day of the week. Sabbath and holiday food should be less heavy and smaller in quantity, conducive to clear thinking and joyful fellowship.

The diet should be prescribed with care particularly for children and pregnant women. Sedentary workers need a diet much lower in fat, sugars, and total calories than do those doing heavy physical work. During the summer, fats and sugars will increase the discomfort experienced because of the heat. Those who are sick can have most of their diseases intelligently treated by the proper selection of the diet. Divine agencies will give skill and understanding to those who put forth efforts to secure a proper diet for the sick. Fresh, new ideas which come as a result of clear mindedness can make a restricted diet palatable and interesting.

Lessons From Nature

Certainly in the introduction of a vegetarian diet, tact and discretion are needed. If the mother in the family stamps her foot down and says: "From this time forth no meat will be served in this home," she may have a rebellion on her hands and may have to retrace her steps. The diet should not be associated in the mind with things unpleasant or oppressive. On the other hand, if she presents a vegetarian meal in a special setting of enjoyment, pageantry, and festivity, such as a birthday, it will be more readily accepted, and may be received as a privileged food.

We should study God's plan for man's food. There were no animal foods in God's original diet for man. The diet designed for him in the Garden of Eden is still best for his needs. Yet, when switching from a diet of animal products, a person may not immediately relish a more wholesome diet. A little perseverance in this matter will be richly rewarded. This kind of diet will recommend itself to thinking people because of its economy, its health-producing qualities, and its simplicity. Office workers often immediately recognize benefits, as do sick persons, and those who have been overworked. Weight control is easier with a vegetarian diet than with any other type of diet. The whole family's needs can be easily supplied by a wholesome diet from grains, fruits, nuts, and vegetables.

A diet that is unpalatable, insipid, or monotonous certainly does not reflect the principles that are taught to us in nature. Our Creator presented the great variety, the assorted array of delightful flavors and aromas, the colors, the shapes, and the consistencies. The lesson taught to us by nature is that it is a false witness against our Heavenly Father if we provide for our families an impoverished, unhappy, and unwholesome dietary, particularly if we then call it health reform.

CHAPTER THREE

Functions of Foods and Food Habits

Why Do We Eat?

Obviously we are composed of what we eat, and what we eat has a profound effect upon our whole being. Foods of the three food groups that should compose the principal part of the menu, (fruits, vegetables, and whole grains) contain 40 to 45 nutrients and various nutrient groups including water and the several gases. Starting with these 40 to 45 nutrients, the body can make literally thousands of substances, some of which are very complex in nature. With these substances, we move, see, hear, speak, taste, remember, feel, smell, think, learn, sing, pray, are creative, and do everything else we are capable of doing. Our understanding is awakened to the fact that proper nutrients make the various functions of the body possible. Without the proper nutrients, none of these functions is possible.

We should learn to think of the various processes of the mind as being as biological as is digestion. Good disposition is due partly to good digestion and nutrition. Good perception and judgment are not happenstance or entirely by virtue of native ability, but rather, as a result of following natural law. "The sin of intemperate eating, eating too frequently, too much, and of rich, unwholesome food, destroys the healthy action of the digestive organs, affects the brain, and perverts the judgment, preventing rational, calm, healthy thinking and acting.... Therefore, in order for the people of God to be in an acceptable state with Him, where they can glorify Him in their bodies and spirits, which are His, they must with interest and zeal deny the gratification of their appetites, and exercise temperance in all things."[79] "People who have a sour stomach are very often of a sour disposition. Everything seems to be contrary to them, and they are inclined to be peevish and irritable. If we would have peace among ourselves, we should give more thought than we do to having a peaceful stomach."[80] Failure to provide for a properly functioning stomach and to observe the laws of health is a "fruitful source of church trials."[81] This causes increased impatience and unhappiness in the family or office and sets the stage for sickness.

John Harvey Kellogg, the finest physician of the last quarter of the 19th century, stated that Horace Fletcher had discovered that thorough mastication of food gradually lessened, and after a time eliminated, the relish for such unwholesome articles as mustard, pepper, and other hot condiments. Even wine taken in small sips, Kellogg said, lost its attraction.

If one chews each bite to a fine cream, the appetite will probably be a safe guide as to quantity of food one should take. Kellogg believed a slight excess of calories to be better than a slight deficiency. We are not certain he was correct in this matter. It may be that the body can reset its metabolic output a little lower more easily than it can strain a little higher. Every possible effort should be made to eat only a sufficient quantity to keep up the strength and barely maintain body weight.

Malnutrition

There are several ways one can be malnourished. Almost invariably when one thinks of malnutrition, he thinks of starvation. In the United States, this is far from the case. Most instances of malnutrition are cases of selective overnutrition. These are either general overnutrition or overnutrition of specific nutrients leading to a condition of imbalance and increased wear and tear. "Our plain food, eaten twice a day, is enjoyed with a keen relish. We have no meat, cake, or any rich food upon our table.... It is seldom I have a faint feeling. My appetite is satisfied. My food is eaten with a greater relish than ever before."[82]

Reasons for malnutrition include a lack of adequate variety or quantity of food, food faddism, social customs, food habits, the use of highly processed and refined foods, ignorance of the basic principles of nutrition, complacency, carelessness, and prejudices developed in childhood (often due to childish whims that are indulged). By very simple means, but often requiring much attention and effort, each of these factors can be eliminated. Since so much is at stake both in the happiness of life and in the productivity for society, it would seem to be more desirable to give these matters our first attention and finest effort. The closer the garden is to the table the more likely the family is to be properly nourished. Instruction in proper selection and preparation of food should be given in every church, every school, and every family.

We have recently begun to recognize overnourishment as a form of malnutrition. Many of our health problems stem from eating too much food, even though of good quality. Eating too freely of certain types of foods such as sugars, caffeinated beverages, animal products, fats, alcohol, spices, vinegar, and salt creates cravings and other difficulties. With the selective overeating of a refined or concentrated food type, there is an imbalance of the nutritional economy which results in a selective undernutrition in another area. "We should not be prevailed upon to take anything into the mouth that will bring the body into an unhealthy condition, no matter how much we like it. Why?-- Because we are God's property.[83] Eating generously of concentrated foods places a strain on the metabolic resources of the body. Certain biochemical systems become clogged at certain points, and the delicate machinery of the human body becomes worn, developing degenerative diseases.

Except in extreme poverty or in food faddism, it is unlikely in our day of efficient transport to have a restricted variety of foods available. The food faddist is likely to restrict his diet in an extreme way along certain specific lines and to overemphasize them. For example, one man, in carrying out his ideas of health reform, daily ordered a bowl of yogurt, an onion, and a slice of whole wheat bread. "Because it is wrong to eat merely to gratify perverted taste, it does not follow that we should be indifferent in regard to our food.... No one should adopt an impoverished diet. Many are debilitated from disease, and need nourishing, well-cooked food. Health reformers, above all others, should be careful to avoid extremes. The body must have sufficient nourishment."[84]

The Hunzakuts living in the Himalaya mountains use a wide variety of fruits, vegetables, berries, whole grains, and seeds. Yet their dietary does not approach the variety used by the average strict vegetarian in the United States. The Hunzakut diet consists mostly of apricots (sun-dried for winter use), vegetables of all kinds, a very small amount of goat's milk, and rarely meat which is eaten on feast days and then only in small amounts. The Hunzakut table will have various platters of raw foods, bowls of cooked vegetables or fruits, and a large bowl of some kind of cooked grain or chapatis. These people are strong and long-lived.

The Akikuyu in Africa eat a restricted diet chiefly of corn and sweet potatoes along with other vegetables. By contrast, the Masai, another African tribe, eat mainly meat and milk and live an average of about 35 years. They are, however, about five inches taller and 23 pounds heavier than the Akikuyu, who live an average of 30 years longer!

It was stated in the *Journal of the American Medical Association*[85] that plant proteins such as legumes and grains "can give...about the same nutritional value as high-quality animal protein foods.... Pure vegetarians from many populations...have maintained seemingly excellent health." Pure vegetarians will do well to provide leafy vegetables as frequently served foods to replace animal products.

Function of Food

Major Nutrients Comprising Foods. Based on their chemical characteristics, there are six major groups of nutrients which make up the foods we eat. All natural foods contain some of all the six groups, but may be more concentrated in one group: legumes are most noted for their protein, peaches for their carbohydrates, etc. The six major nutrients are:

Carbohydrates	Vitamins	Fats
Minerals	Proteins	Water

Fuel Nutrients. Three of the major nutrients (carbohydrates, fats, and proteins) are called "fuel nutrients" as they can be used as sources of energy for various body processes. They must be eaten in large enough quantities to furnish several hundred calories per day. The most economical source of fuel is carbohydrate. The need for fuel varies with exercise and the weather. During heavy exercise and in cold weather, we need more fuel nutrients, but if a day will be spent mainly sitting, normally less fuel will be needed.

Function of food, other than the usually expected ones of bringing longevity and preventing malnutrition, are providing physical stamina, mental alertness, and emotional stability. The quality of diet was shown by Ancel Keys and his co-workers during World War II to be related to work output and behaviour. Food furnishes fuel for energy when oxidized. In order to understand how energy from the sun gets into food, we must understand the following equation of photosynthesis.

PHOTOSYNTHESIS

$$CO_2 + H_2O + Sunlight \xrightarrow[\text{Plant Enzymes}]{\text{Chlorophyll}} CH_2O + O_2$$

$$\text{(Carbon Dioxide)} + \text{(Water)} + \text{(Radiant Energy)} \longrightarrow \text{(Carbohydrates)} + \text{(Oxygen)}$$

Digestion releases the energy stored in the carbohydrates which came originally from the sun. The following equation demonstrates the process of digestion:

DIGESTION

$$CH_2O \text{ (Carbohydrates)} \xrightarrow[\text{B-Complex Vitamins}]{\text{Digestive Enzymes}} \text{Energy} + CO_2 \text{ (Carbon Dioxide)} + H_2O \text{ (Water)}$$

Building Nutrients. Protein, minerals, and water enter tissue composition and can be denoted as "building nutrients." The body has an efficient system which conserves these nutrients so that very little is lost from the processes that use them. Therefore, the body generally needs about the same quantity of each of these three nutrients daily. However, if some special need should arise, such as a burn on the skin, which demands more protein, or excessive sweating which calls for more water, these quantities would need to be increased in proportion to the body's requirements.

Food is utilized as building materials to produce various molecules or portions of molecules to maintain the structure and function of the body, for development of new tissue, and for maintenance of old tissues.

Body Regulators. Minerals and vitamins regulate the various body processes, such as the relaying of messages by nerves (firing of synapses), the clotting of blood, and the formation of new cells. They are known as "body regulators." Generally, just as with the building nutrients, these regulators are needed in about the same quantity daily, but more may be needed during periods of stress. The food substances that must be provided for various processes of the body, such as minerals for muscle contraction and relaxation, transmission of nerve impulses, or the production of digestive juices and enzyme building blocks are called the regulatory nutrients.

Deficiency Diseases

There are several deficiency diseases that are the result of inadequate nutritive elements in the diet. Every cell synthesizes thousands of enzymes. These are proteins of high molecular weight having amazing functions. Vitamins form a part of many enzymes. There are certain enzymes aligned in a very orderly fashion within the mitochondria ("powerhouses") of cells that release energy for the cell. The mitochondria are organelles (small "organs" within a cell) that function in the cell somewhat as lungs function in the body. In this position, the enzymes assist in the utilization of oxygen at a cellular level to produce energy for the cell. This process is called "internal respiration."

It is feared by many that an all-plant diet is marginal or lacking in such nutrients as calcium, iron, riboflavin, vitamin B-12, and vitamin D (for children not exposed to sunlight). However, plant proteins are not to be questioned as being adequate if one judiciously uses combinations of grains that are high in methionine, with legumes that are high in lysine. This demonstrates that diets of properly selected plant foods can be nutritionally adequate.[86] Hardinge and Stare studied 200 vegetarian subjects by physical examination and laboratory analysis and found no evidence of deficiency. Although the B-12 level was judged to be deficient according to understood averages, no cases of anemia were found.

Types of Energy

There are three types of energy obtained from food: kinetic (energy for motion), electrical (cell wall integrity, muscle and nerve impulses), and chemical (manufacture, storage, and transport of chemicals).

Kinetic energy is obtained mainly from the breakdown of carbohydrates in the body, which can be thought of as the reverse of photosynthesis described by the simple equation given earlier. Electrical energy, however, is obtained by a more complex process, as we shall see in a subsequent section. The autonomic nervous system, with its electrical impulses and numerous feedback mechanisms, requires a great deal of energy from foods which must be converted to electrical energy.

Some energy of a chemical nature is also required to supply nerve impulses.

In the regulation of such a complex mechanism as swallowing, literally thousands of impulses must go back and forth between the brain and the esophagus. In swallowing, as in many other processes, all three types of energy are needed. To produce digestants for the release of the energy obtained through photosynthesis, numerous cellular enzymes are called into action. To make these enzymes requires chemical energy. As these enzymes become active, they function to release more chemical energy.

Heat of Specific Dynamic Action

The specific dynamic action of food is the stimulus given to the metabolism mainly by proteins, but also, to a lesser degree, by carbohydrates and fats. A high protein diet stimulates metabolism. This stimulus acts as a tax, not a relief, to the body. Protein in a meal increases the production of heat in the body by about 30%. Carbohydrates and fats increase the body heat production by about 5%. We can see by this differential that protein can easily put a large tax on the body because of its increased metabolic activity. At the same time, one feels stimulated because of the nudge given to the metabolism through the mechanism of the heat of specific dynamic action. This stimulation should not be used as a recommendation for the use of excessive quantities of protein. While the metabolic fires burn hotter with excessive quantities of protein, there is more toxic waste with the subsequent earlier onset of degenerative physical and mental diseases.

Osmotic relationships, antibodies, and plasma globulins are all related to a proper intake of proteins. The use of a high protein diet adds to the burden of the kidneys, the liver, and the gastrointestinal tract. There is a sense of well-being initially observed from a high protein intake due to the stimulus to the metabolism related to the heat of specific dynamic action. On the other hand, many who begin a vegetarian diet mistakenly feel that they are low in protein if they experience a sensation of weakness. While the stimulatory effect of meat and other animal products is lost, there is no actual reduction in muscular strength or endurance—only a sensation of weakness. The sensation usually disappears in about five days. A genuine protein deficiency is accompanied by edema, retardation of growth, wasting of body tissues, weakness, and loss

of vigor.

Food Habits

In various parts of the world, the habits of food preparation or menu planning vary so greatly that they give us a good laboratory to study the influence of food habits on physical health. For example: Many of those who live in the Orient eat mostly vegetables, fruits, and grains while using little in the way of bread or oils. Orientals have very little coronary heart disease on this traditional diet. In Italy, before 1950, breads made up a large portion of the diet, as did legumes. Fried foods occupied only a very small part of the dietary. Since 1950, beer consumption is up 600%, fats 100%, and sugar 200%. These dietary changes have accounted for a threefold increase in obesity among Italians. In America, fats represent the largest single portion of food calories, accounting for about 45% of the total calories obtained from food. Refined carbohydrates represent a large part of the remainder. The influence of this enormous proportion of concentrated nutrients results in accelerated aging, much disability, and death from a variety of degenerative diseases such as coronary heart disease, our number one killer.

In certain selected areas there are isolated traditions involving food items such as breads, pastas, food combinations, etc. These traditions either enhance or reduce the quality of foods served on the table. Every ethnic group has a traditional legume/grain combination. Orientals have rice and soybeans. Latins have *tortillas y frijoles*, Indians have chapatis and garbanzos. Americans have the peanut butter sandwich. Surely this wisdom about the desirability of combining legumes and grains came to the world through inspiration to be a blessing to mankind before the science of nutrition had sufficiently developed to recognize the need for balancing amino acids.

Often the housewife is overly concerned with supplying all the various nutrients her family needs and makes the mistake of putting too many items in the menu. As a result of the complex combinations of chemicals introduced into the stomach, a chemical warfare wages, and nutrients are poorly absorbed or become nonfunctional. Even certain slight but unwanted changes in any one of the three levels of organization in a protein could render that protein nonfunctional. This may come in the form of the alteration of pH, the presence of numerous interfering molecules, or the amount of available water. In addition, many kinds of the R—

groups which project from the protein backbone, or from an individual amino acid, also contain ionizable amino or carboxyl groups (see figure below). These are also capable of acting as bases or acids by picking up or donating protons, respectively, from other available foods. Proteins and amino acids are thus able to act as buffers in cellular and inter-cellular fluids. The simpler the menu, the less interference from conflicting chemicals, and the more beneficial the individual foods.

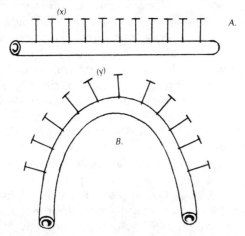

The cylinder represents a rubber tube into which nails have been driven. The nail heads in (a) above are a certain distance, (x), apart when the tube is straight. When the tube is bent, however, the nail heads are spread further apart so that the distance between them is greater, (y). Analogously, the tubing represents the polypeptide backbone and the nails the various amino acid R-groups. If the polypeptide is bent, the distance between the R-groups is changed, affecting the reactivity of the protein. Proteins are very sensitive to certain environmental changes and may become irreversibly altered during the processes of extraction and purification, representing one of the most difficult problems biochemists encounter in their study of proteins.

The most important meal of the day is breakfast. Those who eat a hearty breakfast have fewer accidents and higher performance tests on production, according to industrial statistics. School children get higher grades if they customarily eat a well-balanced breakfast. The best cereal for breakfast is a home cooked cereal such as oatmeal, millet, or farina. Boxed cereals are generally poor. Mapo 30-second Oatmeal, Instant Quaker Oatmeal, Shredded Wheat, and Cheerios take first place in being most nutritious of the ready prepared cereals. Special K, Wheaties, Fruit Loops, and Hearty Granola were found to be fairly nutritious. Least nutritious were found to be Total, Cornflakes, Fruity Pebbles, Corn Chex, and most other boxed cereals.[87]

In every country of the world where food is grown there are natural products that come from the earth that will supply all of the nutrients needed by the individuals who live in that area. Every attempt should be made to encourage every home to have a small garden. It can mean the difference between mediocre health and peak athletic performance.

Instinctive selection of food is not always best. Since tradition, habits, and "Mamma's favorite dish" figure very heavily in the selection of food, some individuals will become undernourished or overnourished if they depend alone on instinctive selection of foods. Malnutrition is still widespread in the world. There are, however, sufficient land and other natural resources to eliminate all hunger from the world, if ignorance and indolence were eliminated, and the greed of a few did not result in extreme inequalities of food distribution.

Cooking and Eating--Science and Art

There is such an art to cooking simply and serving nicely as to make the diners feel that a sumptuous feast has been served. This art of cooking includes blending flavors, choosing consistencies such as crispness and chewiness, and presenting a colorful board. It includes filling the dining area with appetizing odors. The hostess, usually the mother and wife in the home, should preserve a quietness, neatness, and sweet friendliness in the cooking and dining quarters. All boisterousness and unwanted noise is out of place in the dining room. The graciousness of a small plant or a few flowers on the table can change a poor meal into a rich banquet. Most of the things that go to make up the art of cooking and serving are simple and not time consuming. Scrupulous cleanliness in both kitchen and dining room, with strict orderliness, go far in promoting the happiness of the family.

While the art of cooking is the attention to small details, none of which are difficult or expensive, the science of food will require a lifetime of devotion to the study. That may seem to be a large order, but if the student of foods will acquire three good books for only five minutes of study each day, she should be able to become a nutritionist of considerable skill in a couple of years. These three books are a good cookbook such as *Eat for Strength*, a book of nutrition such as this one, and a book explaining the anatomy and physiology of digestion, such as *Counsels on Diet and Foods*. Almost immediately, the new bride can be giving her little family tasty and nourishing meals. She can take pride in her family's zestful living, resistance to disease, good disposition, intelligence, and good looks. The firm, elastic step and the bloom of health on the cheeks are no accident, but are the result of learning and following the rules of good health.

While the art of cooking and serving are worn easily, as a garment, the science of foods represents the skeleton and flesh. The young cook will begin to acquire through study on her own a knowledge of chemistry, physics, human anatomy, and physiology. So easily will the knowledge be obtained, that the pain usually associated with mastering these subjects in academic courses is not felt at all.

The shoulders on which rests the burden of feeding the family should also bear a burden to become informed and trained to do the job well. Before a man marries, he should investigate if the candidate for a wife understands the science of foods and other sciences of health. His future, and that of his children, their health and happiness, and even their eternal salvation may be tied to this one string. It is certainly no blessing to a home to have the mother often cross, frequently sick, or unable to keep the home orderly and clean. Much more depends on her abilities in the kitchen than meets the eye.

There are many telltale indicators of poor eating habits. Being overweight is one sign. Often, the food that person eats is not truly satisfying. It may be too sweet, too soft, too salty or fat. As one gets older, the problem usually gets worse. A brittle temper is often a sign of poor nutrition. Lack of zest for vigorous exercise is another telltale sign. Inability to keep things orderly and clean, fatigue, poor complexion, pallor, soft muscles, and lack of ambition all may stem from poor nutrition. The science of foods will teach one how to put the bloom of youth and the strength of Samson into one's family.

Good food is not expensive. To give an example: A pound of potatoes cooked in the jackets and eaten whole, may cost 20 cents per pound to get ready for serving. Whereas, a pound of potato chips, having lost most of the vitamins and minerals of the fresh potato and having been put through a frying process that may leave traces of carcinogens on the food and add unwanted calories in the form of fat, may cost $1.60 per pound.

Good cooking is not time consuming. The cook should not be required to spend all day in the kitchen, even if she has to gather the food from the garden and prepare it "from the ground up." The more simply our food can be prepared, the more nourishing it will be and, usually, the more flavorful. Each step in processing removes some flavor and nourishment.

Good food tastes and smells good. There are many who feel that in order to be good for one,

food must taste like medicine and leave one with a dissatisfied feeling. Good food is not, in the strict sense medicine, but it will keep you from needing medicine.

Taste buds are of four different varieties, each being stimulated by a different chemical. The taste buds for sweet flavors are located mainly on the tip of the tongue. A chemical having a molecular structure showing a 5-sided ring with a tail is the particular type of chemical structure that will cause one to experience a sweet sensation on the tongue. Seldom will a natural food have only a single one of the four flavor sensations. Most have a distinctive and delightful blend of flavors to give the enormous variety of taste experiences which are possible. By refining, we can separate these tastes into sweet, sour, bitter, and salty. Each of these four sensations is pleasant *if rightly combined*.

Bitter should be so faint as to appear bland in the mouth. Sour should be so correctly combined with another or several flavors as to leave a pleasant experience. No single flavor or texture should be powerful enough that only that flavor and consistency makes the major contribution to the eating experience. Sugar can be such a strong flavor that in order to have any other sensation, concentrated artificial flavoring must be used to salvage the situation. As more and more concentrated flavors are added, the taste quickly becomes perverted and calls for more and more pronounced flavors. We see that one who likes the concentrated and refined flavors of sugar often is a heavy user of salt; or he may be one who enjoys the sharp, strong flavor of tobacco, alcohol, coffee, etc. Bland foods hold no enjoyment for him. He cannot imagine getting pleasure from plain bread; it must be covered with well-salted butter or very sweet jellies or sharp and fatty mayonaise.

If a person as mentioned describes your case, there is good news for you. Before you can believe it is happening, you can begin to relish the delicate, barely perceptible flavors of natural foods. We are now recognizing physical problems in individuals who indulge a perverted appetite for any of the four primary flavors. The appetite is easily trained, and you will be pleased at how soon you will both enjoy natural flavors, and have the satisfaction of knowing you are not damaging your body.

The sour flavors are acid and may damage the teeth on prolonged contact. The sweet foods cause a rise in blood fats and apparently damage the arteries. They also cause a reduction in the ability of white blood cells to engulf bacteria (phagocytic index). Sweets cause tooth decay and deplete the body of vitamin B-1, the good disposition vitamin. Sweets promote fermentation in the stomach and irritate the nerves. Bitter flavors generally come from nicotine, coffee, alcohol, and compounds from the toxic alkaloid group. If bitter flavors are used in foods, they are often sweetened by the use of large quantities of sugar. This can cause abnormal stimulation followed by sedation. Excessive use of salt by population groups produces high blood pressure in people who are susceptible. In Japan, there is 80% more hypertension in the segment of the population using fish pickled in brine, a saturated salt solution.

The cook who is a conscientious student is well-advised to learn to put into each meal foods that will stimulate each of the four flavor sensations. A satisfaction from one's food comes more readily to those whose entire spectrum of taste experiences is stimulated by the meal: sweet, sour, salt, and bland (no bitter). Care should be exercised not to serve too great a variety of food at one meal as the digestive powers are overtaxed by this process.

Influence of Habits on Purchases

Because we are creatures of habit, Americans have gradually, over a period of 75 years, greatly changed their pattern of purchasing. There are some unsettling indications of widespread nutrient deficiencies in certain areas, especially vitamin A and B and iodine. It is a fact that Americans eat too few vegetables and fruits. It is also a fact that they eat too much of the various animal products, too much snack foods, and get overbalanced with fortified foods and food supplements. The food snack is a particularly hazardous area in America. Individuals look and feel well-nourished, because they are plump, strong, and not hungry; and because of their widespread use, many believe the government endorses snack foods. Such is not the case.

Some women have kept family food consumption diaries for several weeks, revealing some very interesting patterns in individual members, as well as in family organization. Dinner is likely to be prepared from convenience and frozen foods and is only fair in nutritional quality. As soon as children come home from school, snacking begins immediately. Most of the foods that are consumed can be classified as "junk" foods--processed snack foods which contain little nutritional value, but kill the appetite for dinner. When dinner is finished, snacking starts about 30 minutes later and continues until bedtime.

The family seldom has time to eat meals, even if mother cooks a well-balanced meal. Mother then feels guilty because she seems to be unable to control things and to perform her duty properly. Therefore, she tends to overspend on certain expensive food items, even if these do not add much to the nutritive value of her meals.

True nutrition education is lacking in our modern way of life. However, there is much anti-nutrition in the form of television advertising, high pressure salesmanship, and clever merchandising of strong aroma, money foods in grocery stores. Conflicting information from authorities about nutrition, scares about such items as pollution, organic gardening, food supplements, vitamins, etc., have all played their part to confuse the issue. It would seem that the fascinating truth about foods and nutrition could be presented at least as interestingly as food advertising on television. All responsible individuals should feel a sense of duty both to learn and to impart information about nutrition to school children and others. Our country can only be as strong as the individuals who compose it.

It is sad, but true, that the committees that study nutrition practices in America often "fall captive to the thiking of the government agencies which contract for their services," according to Phillip M. Boffey, or "as in the case of the Academy's Food Protection Committee, they fall prey to industrial interests." A few years back, the senate appointed an investigation of cereals. The testimony of a prominent American nutritionist before this committee stoutly defended the nutritional benefits of boxed breakfast cereals. How could this nutrition giant be duped into defending breakfast cereals! The answer was simple; he was on the payroll of a large cereal industry to try to upgrade the quality of their inferior product. Any man receiving from ten to twenty thousand dollars yearly from a company is likely to feel somewhat sympathetic toward their interests. Boffey notes that the committee, "has long had very close ties with the food, chemical, and packaging industries which use and produce the chemicals evaluated by the committee." One chairman of the National Academy of Sciences allowed his university research team to receive a research grant from the major producer of monosodium glutamate right in the middle of a research deliberation on the potential hazards of MSG.[88]

CHAPTER FOUR

Growth, Processing, Marketing, and Food Storage

Causes of Large Variation of Nutrients in Foods

There are several ways the nutrient content of foods may be altered. Losses occur in a few nutrients by the leaching of soil and the holding of foods for days or weeks after harvesting. However, the nutrients reduced by soil leaching or long storage can be made up easily, in most cases, by eating a wide variety of foods grown in various geographic areas. The basic rule to insure good nutrition is that of eating a wide variety of fruits, vegetables, whole grains, and nuts, in as natural or unrefined condition as possible. (All other foods and nutrient concentrates should be taken sparingly or avoided altogether.

The really large losses in nutrient content of foods occurs as a result of the reduction of nutrients through hybridization—sometimes 2 or 3 hundred percent reduction. Some vegetables and fruits have been developed to produce a heavy yield without special regard to nutrient content. As an example, over two-thirds of all the nation's green beans are produced in one valley in Oregon. In 1970, a new variety of green beans became available which could be harvested by mechanized equipment. This new variety had not been tested for nutritional content prior to becoming the principle green bean for two-thirds of American families. A new variety of seed can have many-fold more effect on certain nutrients in a given food product than can long, cold storage or any leaching or treatment of the soil.

There are several methods of farming that will insure a superior crop of vegetables and fruits containing adequate amounts of vitamins and minerals. These methods include treatment of the soil, addition of essential minerals and other plant nutrients when needed, selection of the plants and seeds, and techniques of plant culture. If one wishes to obtain the greatest supply of vitamin A, the very best way to do that is to choose foods that develop the greatest quantity of this vitamin during the growth period. Even poor soil will grow sweet potatoes that are high in vitamin A if the proper variety is chosen. There are, however, fifteen times as much vitamin A in the deep, orange-colored sweet potato as in the light yellow sweet potato. The variety of the potato, rather than the quality of the soil, makes the difference. Nevertheless, the type of soil, method of farming (such as hydroponic, row farming, grow boxes with artificial soil, etc.), and the general climatic (especially amounts of sunlight, amounts and timing of watering) and geographic conditions do make some differences in nutrient content. Again, these alterations can usually be compensated for quite easily by following the rule of getting a wide variety from several geographic locations.

Any type of treatment of the soil will make only about a 10% difference in the amount of measurable major nutrients. The really large differences in nutrient content are inherent in the kinds of foods, the kinds of soil or type of fertilization making only slight differences. The yield of the plant is, however, greatly influenced by the quality of the soil that produces the plant, but the measurable content of most nutrients will remain about the same for the same species of plants. To illustrate, let us say that we will use a soil that has only 10% of the calcium needed for optimum growth of a plant. It will produce 10% of the optimum yield. There will be only ten almonds instead of a hundred almonds, but for every hundred grams of those almonds that are produced there will be about 234 mg. of calcium, the normal amount for this particular nutrient.

It seems quite reasonable to assume that there are some nutrients, trace metals, perhaps vitamins, and other unknown nutrients that should be present in food but are unmeasurable by our current technology or are even unknown to our chemists. It may be that these nutrients are of minor importance. On the other hand, they may be of sufficient importance to mean the difference between health and disease. Yet, these nutrients may be absent from the soil, resulting in their absence in the food. Such a nutrient is iodine.

The people living in geographic areas where iodine in the soil is low are more likely to have thyroid disorders such as goiter. The quantity of copper, iodine, and other trace minerals found in vegetables, cereals, and fruits is influenced by the soil content of the minerals. There are certain goiter belts in the interior of the United States which have a lower iodine content in the soil than in seacoast areas.[89] It would appear that continual depletion of the soil, especially if there is heavy farming, soil leaching from heavy rainfall, and replacement of only certain nutrients commercially obtained would make it advisable to add as much compost from rotted vegetable matter as possible. Trace elements present in the recycled plants will thereby be returned to the soil. Likewise, essential minerals, if found to be deficient, should be added.

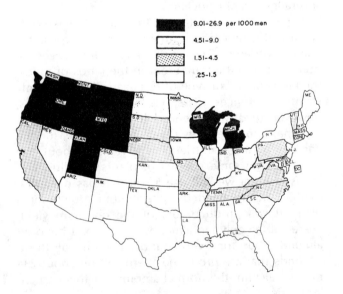

Distribution of simple goiter among drafted men in 1917-1918.

Unsubstantiated Claims for Organic Gardening

Probably nobody would disagree that the natural methods of farming are most desirable for small plots and family gardening. The difficulty with organic methods of farming arises mostly in the area of unscrupulous marketing and unfounded statements. Someone has stated that there are 100 times more organically grown fruits and vegetables sold than the organic farmers produce each year! Often one hears very strong claims about the health-giving properties of organically grown foods. There is often condemnation of foods that are grown on chemically fertilized soils. The word "natural" has a psychological appeal for all of us. One important feature of the "natural" food program is that the soil is the determining factor in the nutrient content of the foods. A frank study of the subject, however, leads one to the conclusion that the variety of plant influences the nutrient content far more than the soil factor.

By careful cross-breeding and selection, researchers have developed a variety of corn that has a much higher content of the amino acid lysine. The same process has produced a tomato which has a higher carotene content than the average tomato. Corn has been developed with an oil content as low as 5%, and another as high as 20%. One type of commercial corn has been bred for its special starch content. A plant produced by research will maintain the desired characteristic no matter what soil it is grown in. The 10% variation due to the soil becomes insignificant, as compared with the variation of nutrients in different varieties of plants, which may be from 20- to 200-fold.

It is sometimes said that the nutrients are higher and pests and diseases are less with organic farming. Experimental evidence seems to tell a different story. In 1938, a study was begun in England which spanned 27 years of experimentation. This study involved two sections of seventy-five acres each. One section was farmed by organic farmers, and the other section was farmed in the ordinary way. In some instances, the organic section proved better, and in some instances, the regular method was better. The overall picture showed no advantage for either method, and all differences were quite small. The chickens grown in the organic section had a loss of two batches due to aspergillosis. There was a complete failure of the kale crop in the organic section. Alfalfa was attacked by wilt in both sections. Wheat in the organic section was attacked by bunt disease. Kale was badly damaged by flea beetles in the organic section.

The question naturally arises: Are commercial fertilizers always harmful to soil or plants? We are convinced that, properly used, they cause little or no trouble. Lightning produces nitrous oxides of the same quality made in factories that produce fertilizers. In the soil, phosphorus is produced by the action of sulfuric acid on phosphate rocks. The sulfuric acid comes from the disintegration of organic matter in the soil. The process is the same as that which goes on in fertilizer factories. Potassium is released from wood ashes, the same potassium compounds as are found in the fertilizer bags. Almost all commercial fertilizers originate from pulverized, treated rock, except for the purely nitrogenous ones which are usually synthetic.

Use Both Methods--
Organic and Non-Organic

Compost will greatly improve the texture and fertility of your soil. It may add certain unmeasurable substances such as trace minerals. It will certainly increase the yields. Humus should be put in the soil to hold moisture and heat, to facilitate ionic exchange between soil and plants, and to provide material to encourage bacterial growth and earthworms. Commercial fertilizers are quite expensive and sometimes difficult to obtain. Harmful pesticides are a hazard. These facts furnish ample reasons for using organic gardening methods as much as possible. However, one should also consider that it is an expensive matter to have a crop failure. It is our opinion that it would be well to treat the soil with the best of both organic and regular methods to insure no crop failures. We should have no fear that we will be undernourished if we use ordinary care in selection, storage, cooking, serving, and chewing of our food.

It is true that the earth has been leached of many of its nutrients and that plants are grown in soil that lacks certain vital nutrients. Some foodstuffs which should contain minerals or other complexes do not have as complete a supply of nutrients as those grown in the very best of soils. In the time before the flood, plants grew to giant sizes, were resistant to diseases, and had beautiful symmetry and loveliness in all ways. Now the plants are suffering under the same curse of degenerative processes that involve men. "The earth shall wax old like a garment."[90] Nevertheless, with our own diminutive size and our less active metabolic processes, the earth produces sufficiently well to supply our smaller nutritional needs. We should remember the promise that the Lord made to Noah: "While the earth remaineth, seedtime and harvest, and cold and heat, and summer and winter, and day and night shall not cease."[91]

Processing of Food

Food processing robs foods of many of their vital nutrients. Since losses in nutrient content have occurred at various points in production of food, it is of vital importance that we not allow major losses at the time of food processing. We can reduce the content of some nutrients in food by rinsing or soaking in water after cutting, peeling, snapping, or shredding. Foods such as chopped lettuce, snapped beans, peeled Irish potatoes, and any other vegetables that have been pared or broken in any way should not be soaked in water after having been cut. To do so causes significant losses of water soluble vitamins and minerals. Even flavor is lost. It is possible to destroy certain nutrients that are labile to heat and light and remove others that are sensitive to aging, oxidation, etc. Many nutrients can be reduced to zero by improper handling. If a particular food is expected to provide quite a sizable portion of certain nutrients such as vitamin C or thiamine, and these are lost in processing, the loss may have serious consequences in terms of reduction of constitutional strength or mental efficiency.

There are avoidable dangers in the processing of food aside from the loss of nutrients and the addition of injurious chemicals. The cooking process can represent another hazard. Some people are sensitive to gas used as a fuel in kitchen stoves. They may suffer from headaches or other physical symptoms. Some develop nerve or emotional symptoms as a result of exposure to gas fumes. All people are apparently more susceptible to bronchial irritations if they live in a home having a gas stove. We recommend, as more healthful, an electric stove. Wood cook stoves are of course healthful, but are seen rarely today.

Another potential hazard is the microwave oven. While there is no conclusive evidence to show that using microwave ovens will increase one's risk of cancer or other diseases, there is also no conclusive evidence showing that they are safe. There are some indications, however, that exposure to microwaves may pose a cancer risk. Microwave ovens can leak nonionizing radiation if the door interlock system, which turns the oven off when the door is opened, is poorly adjusted. The FDA has issued a leakage standard of five microwatts per square centimeter at five centimeters from the oven surface for the lifetime of ovens manufactured after October 6, 1971. No one knows, however, if this standard is safe. It is recommended that persons stay at least two feet away from the oven while it is on.[92] Certainly the prudent course is for pregnant women and children to keep their distance until these very convenient appliances have been proven through 20-30 years of wide use to be entirely safe.

Marketing

"Nicely prepared vegetables and fruits in their season will be beneficial, if they are of the best quality, not showing the slightest sign of decay, but are sound and unaffected by any disease or decay."[93] Diseases produced by decayed produce are degenerative in nature, as well as infectious and irritative. A Mississippi researcher named Ford ran some experiments in the early sixties showing that animals fed decayed vegetable matter suffered more from both cancer and heart disease than controls fed fresh feed. When the animals were slaughtered and fed to a second test group, the same tendency to produce cancer and atherosclerosis existed. It apparently did not matter whether the animals got the fermented food first or second hand.

Marketing of foods usually causes some loss of nutrients due to improper storage, long delays between gathering and marketing, overheating, wilting, drying, bruising, etc. All of these take their toll in the food value of the final product. Nevertheless, despite the long distance covered between the garden and the table and improper methods of storage, there are sufficient nutrients remaining in foods to meet nutritional needs. This necessitates that we use care to follow the primary rule of nutrition--taking a wide variety of unrefined foods.

There are several faulty methods of food storage that result in highly significant losses of nutrients from the individual parts. Allowing a long exposure to sunlight in field or orchard, storing at too high a temperature, or storing in an area having too high or too low a moisture content can cause nutritional loss. Especially when foods are chopped or broken in any way, oxidation, light exposure, and moisture content of air may all cause heavy losses of certain nutrients. The storage of canned foods results in smaller losses of fragile nutrients if the storage temperature is nearer to 50 degrees than to 75 degrees.

Autolytic Enzymes

In all raw foods, there are "autolytic enzymes" that automatically begin to destroy the foods as soon as they are cracked, broken, cut, or bruised in any way. These enzymes serve the desirable function of bringing a stabilization in the ecology. If it were not for them, foods and other vegetation that were spoiling would remain in a state of partial decay on the surface of the earth far longer than they do. Autolytic enzymes bring about recycling more rapidly than is possible without them.

This speeding up of the self-destructive process so beneficial in one area will work against us in another way. They also result in some difficulty in maintaining the nutritional value of the foods that are being prepared for the table. In order to avoid the self-destruction mechanism, certain precautions must be observed. Handle fruits and vegetables very carefully, since bumping, squeezing, or bruising may release the autolytic enzymes. When food is being prepared for cooking, it is desirable to heat the water to a vigorous boil *before* the vegetables are added. In this way, autolytic enzymes are inactivated quickly. Most of these enzymes are destroyed by near boiling temperatures. It is this feature that makes blanching of some vegetables before freezing important. The activity of many autolytic enzymes is greatly retarded by freezing, but destroyed only by heating. Since storage in very low temperatures, between -20 degrees and 0 degrees Fahrenheit—retards the enzymes that bring about destruction or ripening of fruits and vegetables, these low temperatures will prevent the loss of flavor, discoloring, and development of strong flavors in frozen vegetables.

Low temperatures also prevent rancidity from developing in the fats which are present in grains, nuts, and seeds. It is wise to keep whole grain flours and other ground or cracked grains at refrigerator or freezer temperature to retard rancidity. The activity of some enzymes is not sufficiently retarded by freezing to prevent the development of a strong or unpleasant flavor in the food. For these foods, blanching can improve the appearance, flavor, and consistency of the finished product. Blanching raises the temperature of the food high enough to denature the enzymes, destroying this activity.

Cooked food gradually develops nitrites if it is not stored at refrigerator temperatures. Nitrites are capable of combining with amines in the intestinal tract to form nitrosamines. These substances are cancer-producing. It is felt that one reason that the United States has seen an unexpected decline in cancer of the stomach in the past fifty years may be due to the widespread practice of refrigeration of leftover foods. Before the era of refrigerators in every home, leftovers were kept at room temperature, which promoted the production of nitrates and nitrites.

Canning is a good way to preserve the excess food grown during the months of heavy garden and orchard production. There is some nutrient loss of fragile vitamins, but the variety of foods eaten at the typical American table more than compensates for the nutrient losses. The method of canning makes a difference. A simple waterbath is sufficient for fruits and acid vegetables, such as tomatoes. All other vegetables must be processed by pressure canner if they are to be properly preserved. Botulism can develop from improperly processed vegetables, meats, and nuts. Botulism results in sudden death soon after eating of the toxic food. Unfortunately, the toxins cannot be seen, smelled, or tasted. Fortunately, the toxin can be destroyed by heat.[94] Boiling for 20 minutes will render home canned vegetables safe. With each waterbath type canner or pressure canner comes a booklet with proper instructions for procedures which have been worked out by trial and error and will give the best results if properly followed. It is not necessary to add either salt or sugar to vegetables or fruits for preserving. Actually germs will probably grow even better if the usual teaspoon per quart of salt or sugar is added, as that small amount merely enriches the culture medium, but is nowhere near the quantity required for preserving food by chemical inhibition of bacterial growth.

It can be seen that the health, happiness, and longevity of the family are very intimately associated with small details of preparing, cooking, and storing of food. No woman should even contemplate marriage until she has mastered the art of healthful cooking; and conversely, any man who is seeking a wife, should make sure that she is a good cook. "Every woman who is at the head of a family and yet does not understand the art of healthful cookery should determine to learn that which is so essential to the well-being of her household....She... should put herself under the instruction of some good cook, and persevere in her efforts for improvement until she is mistress of the culinary art."[95]

CHAPTER FIVE

CARBOHYDRATES

The Best Fuel for the Body

The number of organic fuels that can be taken into the system is partly controlled by the availability of enzymes. If too many different types of nutrients are presented to the system, a war wages inside because of competition among the various chemicals. The enzymes attach to the organic fuels in such a way that there is a competition for entry into the chemical cycles for the breakdown of nutrients to release energy (catabolism cycles). During the delay occasioned by the war, fermentation products accumulate, are absorbed into the blood, and toxicity develops manifested by headache, mental dullness, restlessness, cravings, or irritability.

Another determinant of the number of organic fuels entering the catabolism cycle is the particular type of organic fuels. A greater proportion of glucose can be taken than of fructose. Fructose can be taken in greater proportion than galactose, and galactose greater than Arabinose. There is an ideal balance. From this it can be readily recognized that concentrated food supplements put into the organic fuel cycles in large quantities can clog the machinery. Nutrients come more balanced from natural foods than from nutrient concentrates.

The third limiting factor in the amount of food processed through the catabolism cycles is the amount of oxygen available. There is a maximum amount of oxygen available for catabolism. Many years ago the Pasteur effect was discovered while working with microorganisms. When deprived of oxygen, yeasts were observed to form fermentation products. It was subsequently demonstrated that the Pasteur effect takes place in most mammalian tissues. When the catabolism system is deprived of oxygen, we begin to form fermentation products.

Some of these fermentation products are alcohols, aldehydes, amines, esters, and a number of other toxins. We can have a deficiency of oxygen from two causes: first, insufficient air taken via the lungs into the blood, perhaps from lung disease, impure air, bad posture, or shallow breathing; second, from insufficient or inefficient delivery of oxygen-rich blood to the tissues. Reasons for the decreased blood flow include atherosclerotic narrowing of vessels, "hardening of the arteries" from hypertension, and shunting of blood flow away from vital structures due to reflex mechanisms (chilling of extremities, overeating, lack of exercise, emotional stress, or tight clothing).

What are Carbohydrates?

Carbohydrates are the most abundant and economical sources of energy available in the world today. Because of their abundance, we can expect that foods high in carbohydrates will be very important in preventing starvation as overpopulation mounts. The present emphasis on high protein foods such as meats, milk, and cheese would end abruptly were these products no longer commercially available. We can provide a balanced dietary from the low-cost foods available in most countries. When forced by circumstances to do so, nutritionists learn to balance menus using the native products. As the high protein foods become less and less available, we will find that carbohydrates can form much more than the current 60% of the daily American dietary with good results. These carbohydrates should be unrefined or "complex carbohydrates;" that is, carbohydrates associated with a full native complement of minerals, vitamins, proteins, and fats.

We recognize the ideal in nutrient balance as

more than 60% carbohydrates, less than 15% protein, and less than 20% fat. At the present time in America, we average more than 45% of our dietary calories in the form of fats. In one recent survey it was 50%! In the Orient, approximately 80% of calories come from complex carbohydrates; in the tropics, up to 90% or more. Probably the ideal diet for Americans would contain about 70-80% of the calories as carbohydrates, 10-20% as fat, and 8-10% as protein. When cooking techniques are improved to the point that plain bread can be taken with relish, there will be no reluctance to accept meals so simply and naturally prepared.

Foods for fuel to produce energy can be carbohydrates, fats, or proteins, but carbohydrates make by far the best fuel. Carbohydrates are the cheapest and most readily available source of energy on this planet. They are readily digested and are, of course, the most efficient and rapidly obtainable sources of energy. No part of the carbohydrate molecule is left over to be disposed of in some way other than through the process that furnishes energy. Athletes and physical laborers understand clearly that we get energy easiest from carbohydrates, not from fats and proteins! There are leftover products in the metabolism of both fats and proteins that make them less favorable as energy sources. Carbohydrates can be used under anaerobic conditions as when muscular activity outstrips the ability of the lungs to keep up with oxygen supply. The body tends to conserve carbohydrate for brain function and uses fat for usual activity when under conditions of food deprivation.

Physical exercise does not significantly increase the need for protein. Cross-country skiers who raced 20-50 miles in one day were compared with resting athletes used as controls to determine if the active athletes used more protein. It was found that there was no appreciable difference in the amount of protein used between the two groups.

Furthermore, of the three major classes of nutrients—carbohydrates, fats, and proteins--carbohydrates are by far the most abundant in nature. All natural foods contain some portion of each of these three nutrients but in widely differing proportions. Carbohydrates get their name from their molecular composition, carbon and water. Hydrogen and oxygen maintain the same 2:1 ratio as in water, hence the portion of the word "hydrate."

The caloric requirements of an individual will vary with the type of activity generally performed. Sedentary activity uses approximately 0.23 calories per pound of body weight per hour. Light to moderate exercise uses approximately 0.27 to 0.50 calories, while more active exercise such as fast walking uses 0.77. Strenuous exercise, including swimming, running, and very heavy work, uses 1.09.

Another method of determining energy expenditure is by figuring the number of calories used per minute. Walking at 2.5 miles per hour uses about 3.5 calories per minute; cycling at 5.5 miles per hour uses 4.5; walking at 3.75 miles per hour uses 5.6; horseback riding (trotting) uses 8; cycling at 13 miles per hour uses 11; and running at 10 miles per hour uses 15. A fifteen-minute run would use about 225 calories (15 calories per minute for 15 minutes).

The general formula for carbohydrates is CH_2O: one molecule of water for each carbon atom. The composition of carbohydrates is simple. Monosaccharides have one sugar molecule; disaccharides have two; oligosaccharides have three to ten; and polysaccharides have up to 10,000 or more. The monosaccharides include chiefly two sugars–the sugar of blood, or glucose, which comes from grapes, corn, fruit, roots, and honey; and fructose, which comes from fruits.

Disaccharides are such sugars as sucrose (common table sugar), which is composed of glucose and fructose, and comes mainly from cane and beets; maltose, composed of glucose linked to glucose, comes from barley; and lactose, present only in milk, is glucose linked to galactose. Polysaccharides are starch, dextrins, cellulose, glycogen, and inulin (composed of links of a monosaccharide).

Starch grains may contain as many as 1,300 individual glucose units. Amylase is required for the digestion of starch. Maltose, a disaccharide, requires another enzyme, maltase, to split the disaccharide maltose into the monosaccharide glucose. Galactose is converted by galactase to glucose. Lactose is a combination of glucose and galactose.

"It is not good to eat much honey...."[96] "Hast thou found honey? Eat so much as is sufficient for thee, lest thou be filled therewith, and vomit it."[97] These quotes indicate that the ancients were not accustomed to eating much honey. Honey is at least 70% sugar by law; 29% fructose, 29% glucose, and 12% sucrose, as a minimum. Such a concentrated food should be taken very sparingly.

The central nervous system uses glucose most efficiently as a source of fuel, but can use small amounts of intermediate compounds. Glycogen is formed of linked molecules of glucose. The brain should have a ready source of glucose available in proper quantities for the most perfect functioning.

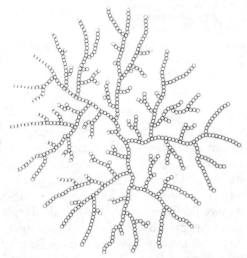

Glycogen: Each round unit represents a glucose molecule.

Fructose, in the blood or in spoiled fruit in the kitchen, is converted to lactic acid upon utilization in the biochemical systems of plants or animals. When an excess of fructose appears in the blood, it is converted to lactic acid. Some physiologists associate lactic acid build-up in muscles with the appearance of symptoms of fatigue. Fructose seems to be more difficult for the biochemical systems to handle than glucose. It skips certain steps in Kreb's cycle of energy production, and may clog the cycle down the line, especially if there is some impairment of liver function. Fifty centimeters of jejunum can absorb eight grams per hour of glucose but only five grams per hour of fructose.

Relative sweetness of various sugars can be tabulated as follows:

Sugar	Sweetness
Honey	120
Fructose	110-175
Sucrose	100
Sorbitol	100
Mannose	100
Glucose	75
Galactose	35-70
Dextrins	30
Lactose	15-30
Starch	5

Uses of Carbohydrates

Energy. In the body, the reverse of the photosynthetic process yields energy with carbon dioxide and water as by-products. Carbon dioxide is breathed off in the lungs, and water is used to hydrate the tissues or is eliminated through the kidneys.

Protein Sparing. If sufficient carbohydrates are present in the diet, very little protein needs to be taken in. If there is a short supply of carbohydrates, proteins will be utilized for energy, but inefficiently, leaving over some parts of the protein molecule that cannot be converted to energy. Approximately 58% of the amino acid molecules stored in the body, and approximately 10% of fat molecules stored in the body can be converted to energy. The remnants of the molecules of both amino acids and fats must be dealt with as waste matter in the biochemical systems. It can be readily appreciated that using these nutrients for fuel comes with a surcharge already fixed, and must not be largely used for fuel if optimum efficiency is to be maintained. These left-over parts place a tax on the kidneys, liver, and other organs to dispose of them. Sometimes the left-over portions are toxic to joints, arteries, nerves, and brain. Degenerative diseases such as arthritis, senility, atherosclerosis, malignancies, and shortened lifespan in experimental animals have been shown to be the result of overeating protein.

Fat Metabolism. In order to prevent the build-up of ketone bodies when fats are metabolized, carbohydrates must be available for attachment. If there is not sufficient carbohydrate, fat metabolism cannot proceed efficiently and an acid condition develops from the ketone bodies.

Antitoxic Effect. Carbohydrates combine with certain toxic chemical by-products of digestion, and bacterial action assists in preventing toxic build-ups. For this reason, the generous use of carbohydrates in the diet can offer an important protective mechanism to the body. A number of vegetables have been tested and shown to counteract many of the toxic effects of drugs, chemicals, and food additives such as Red II dye and cyclamates. The protective effect is more than can be accounted for on the basis of cellulose, and probably involves other plant fibers such as lignins, gums, pectins, mucilages, and hemicelluloses. Many leafy vegetables, grasses, psyllium seed, agar, gum guar, water cress, parsley, celery, carrots, and others have been tested.[98]

Energy for Nerve Tissues. Carbohydrates represent almost the entire source of energy for nerve tissue, as fats and proteins cannot be utilized well by nerve cells to produce energy.

Laxative Action and Normal Peristalsis. Digestible, unrefined carbohydrates are usually accompanied by much indigestible fiber which is bulky in the colon and causes the colon to have more normal function. Cellulose and other long-chain, indigestible carbohydrates such as hemicellulose, gums, pectin, etc., function to help the colon have better health. These polysaccharides stimulate peristalsis in all parts of the bowel, particularly in the colon. They absorb water, thereby giving bulk to the contents of the bowel, causing a more active peristaltic movement. If the digestible carbohydrates pass through the small bowel without being completely digested and absorbed, they ferment in the colon, producing irritating acids and gas. While their presence in the colon is undesirable, they are capable of giving a laxative action.

Precursor Substances. The carbohydrates furnish many vital molecular parts for cells. Carbohydrates are active in the formation of various cellular chemicals such as nucleic acid, the phosphosugars, and certain parts of fatty substances of the blood (triglycerides, etc.). Carbohydrates also act as precursors of many other vital elements such as enzymes, hormones, and parts of cells.

Only a limited quantity of carbohydrates in the form of glycogen can be stored in the body. Glycogen, the animal equivalent of starch, comprises about 6% of the weight of the liver; whereas muscle contains about 0.7%.

If one takes large quantities of carbohydrates, the excess is converted mainly to fat and stored in the adipose tissue depots. The refined carbohydrates cause tooth decay. Experimental animals fed a carbohydrate-free diet or a diet in which the carbohydrates are administered to the stomach via tube do not develop dental caries.

Successful absorption of nutrients from the small bowel is dependent on several factors: (1) The various kinds of starch grains have a distinct granular structure, specific for the particular grains and legumes in

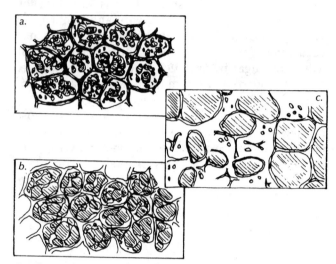

Starch granules: a. Raw; b. Cooked; c. Thoroughly cooked. *(Adapted from Bogert, Briggs, and Calloway. NUTRITION AND PHYSICAL FITNESS, 8th ed., W.B. Saunders Co., 1966, p. 24)*

which they occur. Some granules are more resistant to digestion than others. Long cooking is needed to soften and break down the starch granules for easy assimilation. "Grains used for porridge or 'mush' should have several hours cooking"[99] Monosaccharides require no digestion in the intestinal tract. Very small amounts are absorbed from the stomach. (2) Glucose enters the cell membrane through a "carrier" system as does sodium. These two nutrients seem somewhat interdependent. The availability of the carrier system determines glucose absorption to some degree; therefore, hormone balance, especially of adrenal and pituitary hormones which govern sodium ion exchange, is important to glucose absorption. (3) The mixture of foods in the small intestine determines to some degree the rate of absorption of glucose. Generally, the more simple the meal and the fewer kinds of food eaten, the more easy and complete are absorption and digestion. Another factor determining the rate of absorption is the existence of inflammation or irritation. Depending on the location and nature of the inflammation, nutrients may be either hastened or hindered in their absorption. (4) Too great a variety or quantity of food, however well masticated, will result in a competition for absorption sites at the intestinal mucosa and for the utilization of other transport systems. "It would be much better to eat only two or three different kinds of food at a meal than to load the stomach with many varieties....So many varieties are introduced into the stomach that fermentation is the result. This condition brings on acute disease, and death frequently follows."[100] It is likely that some of the coronary heart attacks and strokes that follow large meals have their origins in this mechanism. The availability of B-vitamins also influences the rate at which carbohydrates and sugars are absorbed.

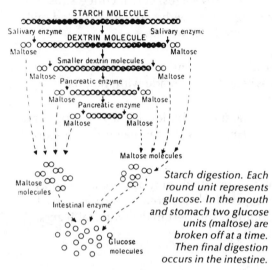

Starch digestion. Each round unit represents glucose. In the mouth and stomach two glucose units (maltose) are broken off at a time. Then final digestion occurs in the intestine.

(Adapted from Bogert, Briggs, and Calloway. NUTRITION AND PHYSICAL FITNESS, 8th ed., W.B. Saunders Co., 1966, p. 360)

Blood Sugar

There are many factors that influence the level of glucose in the blood: the intake of food, the physical and chemical make-up of foods (e.g., refinement), hasty eating causing unstable blood glucose in patients with maturity onset diabetes,[101] physical activity and energy expenditures as from exercise or chilling, and the activity of various hormones: insulin and glucagon from the pancreas, adrenalin from the adrenals, and the respective hormones from the thyroid and pituitary.

Bread, the great "staff of life" in nearly every country, is an excellent source of carbohydrates. Bread may be either unleavened bread or yeast bread. There are several cookbooks such as our Eat for Strength, that have good sections on unleavened breads. There are crackers using no baking soda or baking powder (which are unhealthful) or yeast. Yeast breads include such things as loaves and rolls. There are good recipes for wheat thins, sesame thins, graham crackers, etc., all without leavening.

Granola made with honey has less lysine available than granola made with sugars not having free fructose. Apparently during the browning process, the fructose in honey reacts with lysine to bind it and make it unavailable for absorption. The browning is called the "Maillard reaction." In one experiment, rats grew at only one-third the rate if they were fed granola made with honey than those fed granola made with other sweeteners. It is assumed that zwieback made from bread baked with honey would show a similar effect. We recommend granola made without sweeteners as the original recipes outlined, and is still done in many places, such as Australia.

Because of the great increase in the use of fats, the total carbohydrate intake in the United States has, during the past 60 years, decreased by almost 25%. However, the consumption of sugars and syrups has increased during that same period of time by 25%! The decreased consumption of flour, cereals, and potato products has accounted for the decline. Notice that in these foods the important complex carbohydrates are found. The highly beneficial effects of carbohydrates, such as the antitoxic action, assistance in fat metabolism, energy for nerve tissue, protein sparing, and laxative action are largely lost by these two factors—1) reduction in total intake, and 2) increase in refined carbohydrate use. Not the least of the good factors lost is economy, both in outlay in money for food and in the expense to the body systems.

Sugar yields about four calories per gram, proteins about four, fats about nine, and ethyl alcohol approximately seven. About 50% of the calories of the world are provided from cereals which are composed of approximately 75% carbohydrate, 10-15% protein, and 2% fat. The protein of the germ of cereal grains is of high quality, but the germ is usually removed from wheat, rice, and corn before marketing to prevent early rancidity, increase shelf life, and decrease the economic losses due to spoilage. In the endosperm of the grain, there is another protein, gluten, of not such high biologic value as that in the germ. Some individuals may have an intolerance for gluten. The gluten-free diet is here presented for the benefit of these persons.

Gluten-Free Diet

Gluten is found in wheat, oats, barley, rye, malt, and in many prepared products. Labels must be carefully read. It is not found in millet, rice, or corn. Here is a general diet to help you avoid gluten.

Gluten Free Diet

	Foods Allowed	**Foods Not Allowed**
Beverage	Water; fruit juices; herb teas; Milk substitutes	Alcoholic Beverages; cereal coffee substitutes; beverage made with chocolate; malted milk, drinks made with malt.
Bread	Breads and muffins made with corn, potato, rice, soybean, millet.	Breads made from barley, buckwheat, oats, rye, or wheat; breads made with malt flavoring or extract.
Cereal	Corn and rice cereals without malt flavoring or extract; millet; popcorn (without oil, best for cereal.)	Any made from barley, buckwheat, oats, rye, or wheat; any with malt flavorings or extract.
Dessert	Vegetarian gelatin desserts, fruit puddings, (cornstarch, rice, tapioca, arrowroot starch) fruit smoothies; sweet potato and butternut squash desserts, carob, and coconut.	Desserts made from foods not allowed as cakes, cookies, ice cream, pastries, pies, puddings, sherbert made with stabilizers.
Fat	Cooking fats; fortified margarine; Oils; no more than 15 gm (1 tablespoon) daily; nuts, olives, peanut butter.	Cream, commercial salad dressings made from foods not allowed.
Fruit	Any juice; banana; grapefruit or orange; canned or cooked apples apricots, cherries, peaches, pears, puree of cranberries, dried fruits, and plums.	
Potato or Substitute	White potato; rice; soy spaghetti (if not made with grains).	Fried potato, potato chips, sweet potato, hominy, macaroni, noodles, spaghetti.
Soup	Fat-free broth or bouillon; vegetable soup made from foods allowed; fruit soup; chowders.	Soups made from foods not allowed.
Sweets	Honey; molasses; syrup.	Candy, jam, and marmalade made from foods not allowed.
Vegetables	Any juice; lettuce, raw tomato, cooked asparagus, beets, carrots, pumpkin, squash, string beans, tomatoes, puree of corn, lima beans, peas, puree of spinach.	
Miscellaneous	Salt, herbs, lemon juice; garlic; chives; onion.	Chocolate, gravy; malt extract or flavoring; pickles, white sauce, spices.

Adapted from Mayo Clinic Diet Manual, Third Edition, Philadelphia: W. B. Saunders

High Fiber Diet

Crude fiber represents cellulose and lignin. Bran is almost entirely cellulose. Other indigestible carbohydrates, all being polysaccharides, include algal, hemicelluloses, gums, pectins, and mucilages. In recent years, much has been written about the advantages of a high fiber diet. Dr. Denis Burkitt has done more to publicize the need for a high fiber diet than anyone since Sylvester Graham. Many human diseases are associated with a low intake of total dietary fiber: constipation, colon cancer, diverticulosis, polyposis coli, hemorrhoids, varicose veins, heart and artery disease, and diabetes. The application of the general rule of nutrition, "a wide variety of foods, taken in as natural a state as possible" would eliminate most of our problems with fiber.

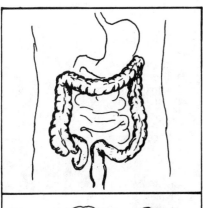

Normal colon.

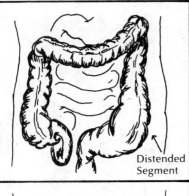

Atonic constipation due to weak muscular activity. Note the distended descending and sigmoid colon.

Distended Segment

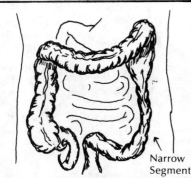

Spastic constipation due to a narrowed segment of descending colon.

Narrow Segment

Sugar Causes Problems

The list of physical and mental disorders related to sugar is formidable. Free sugar has been shown to reduce the ability of white blood cells to function properly, to aggravate heart disease, to reduce life-span, and to contribute to alcoholism, mental illness, high blood pressure, skin diseases, and enlarged liver and kidneys. Many processed cereals contain up to 60% sugar and should be classified as "junk foods." If sugar and water are taken together, the sugar markedly reduces the rate of stomach emptying and therefore reduces the rate at which fluid can be delivered to the intestine for absorption. It is clear, then, that soft drinks, cold fruit juices, and other sweet, cold drinks are not as healthful, nor can they cure dehydration as efficiently as plain, cool water.

Dr. Donald Davis, a University of California chemist, found that rats fed a diet of sugar and processed foods developed a 50% greater appetite for sugar and an 18% greater craving for alcohol than rats fed a similar diet supplemented with twelve vitamins and thirteen minerals. A huge appetite for sweets could be the body's signal that it is nutritionally deprived.

If sugar is completely burned, some of the molecules, such as pyruvic acid, accumulate in the brain, leading to mental dullness. Tooth decay is influenced more by refined carbohydrates than by any other single dietary item. At the age of two years, one of every two babies already has a decayed tooth. Whole grains enhance the resistance against caries.

Chromium, known to be important in pancreatic function, is removed from the diet by sugar refining and by the milling of wheat. Vegetables high in protein tend to have good chromium levels. The milling of wheat into refined white flour removes 40% of the chromium, 86% of the manganese, 76% of the iron, 89% of the cobalt, 68% of the copper, 78% of the zinc, and 48% of the molybdenum. These are trace elements essential for life or health.

Yemenite Jews living in Israel for more than 25 years have a significant increase in atherosclerosis, heart disease, and diabetes. These diseases were extremely rare before moving to Israel where fats are mainly of animal origin and carbohydrates are largely refined. In Yemen, carbohydrates are derived almost solely from fruits, grains, and vegetables, with little sugar; their former diets were also high in fiber and pectins which reduce cholesterol and do not produce rapid increases in blood sugar after meals.

Some studies designed to determine the effect of certain nutrients such as sugar on the movement and activity of white blood cells have revealed many matters of interest. As glucose levels in the blood rise, gram-positive bacteria grow better in blood. Defects were found in the movements of certain white blood cells, called neutrophils, in rheumatoid arthritis, diabetes, and malignancies. These white blood cells increase in numbers in the blood stream when the body has a bacterial infection. These cells normally destroy bacteria. They are the body's soldiers. However, when the blood sugar level goes up, these cells get sluggish and cannot destroy as many bacteria. Chemotaxis (migration of white blood cells toward a chemical attraction such as germs) was less in 24 patients with rheumatoid arthritis. Phagocytosis, the process of eating by the cell, may be normal in these patients, but the cells simply cannot move easily from place to place. Increased sugar intake elevates the serum lipoprotein levels, which is just as bad, if not worse than a high cholesterol in the production of heart disease. Sugar has the ability to stimulate the production of fat in the body in some way apart from its caloric content in the diet. The stimulating effect of sugar appears to be particularly enhanced by the presence of hormonal substances such as those found in "the pill."

Effect of Sugar Intake on Ability of White Blood Cells to Destroy Bacteria

Amount of sugar eaten at one time by average adult in teaspoons	Number of bacteria destroyed by each WBC	Percentage decrease in ability to to destroy bacteria
0	14	0
6	10	25
12	5.5	60
18	2	85
24	1	92
Uncontrolled Diabetic	1	92

Hidden Sugar in Familiar Foods

	Measure	Equivalent Teaspoons sugar
Candies		
Butterscotch candy	1 piece (5 gm or 1¼ tsp.)	1
Chewing gum	1 piece (3gm)	½
Fudge	1 oz. square (28gm)	4
Hard candy	1 piece (5gm)	1
Hershey candy	1 small bar (41gm)	5
Marshmallow	1 average	1½
Peanut brittle	1 piece (25mg)	3½
Cakes and Cookies		
Angel food	1/10 average cake (45gm)	5½
Chocolate cake (iced)	1 piece (85gm)	5½-8
Chocolate chip cookie	1 (11gm)	1½
Doughnut (glazed with jelly center)	1 (65gm)	6
Sandwich type cookie	1 (14gm)	2
Beverages		
Beer	8 oz. (240gm)	2
Chocolate milk	8 oz. (240gm)	5-6
Chocolate milkshake	8 oz. (240gm)	10-12
Cola drinks	6 oz. (one bottle) (180gm)	3½-4
Wine, port	3½ oz. (100gm)	3
Desserts		
Apple pie	1 slice (160gm)	12
Banana split		24
Cherry pie	1 slice (160gm)	12
Hot fudge sundae	1 dish (266gm)	16-17
Chocolate pudding	½ cup (144gm)	6-7
Custard	½ cup (112gm)	4
Gelatin (sweetened)	½ cup (120gm)	4½
Ice cream	½ cup (67gm)	3
Lemon meringue pie	1 piece (140gm)	10½
Sherbet	½ cup (96gm)	5-6
Strawberry shrotcake	1 serving (175gm)	12
Syrups, Sugars, Snacks		
Brown sugar	1 tablespoon (14gm)	2½-3
Honey	1 tablespoon (20gm)	3½
Jam, jelly	1 tablespoon (20gm)	3
Maple syrup	1 tablespoon (20gm)	2½
Sweet pickle	1 large (100 gm)	7½
Fruits		
Apricots, dried	4 to 5 halves (25gm)	3
Dates, pitted	5 (50gm)	7
Figs, dried	2 small (30gm)	4
Grape juice (unsweetened)	½ cup (120gm)	4
Grapefruit juice (unsweetened)	½ cup (125gm)	2
Orange juice	½ cup (124mg)	2½
Peaches, canned	2 halves	3½
Prunes, dried	2 large (20gm)	3
Prune juice	½ cup (120gm)	4-4½
Raisins	1 tablespoon (10gm)	1½
Bread and Cereals		
Cinnamon bun	1 average (97gm)	10½
Cheerios	1 cup (25gm)	3½
Cornflakes, Wheaties	1 cup (22-28gm)	4-4½
Doughnut	glazed	8
Hamburger bun	1 whole bun (30gm)	3
Hot dog bun	1 whole bun (36gm)	3½
White bread	1 slice (23gm)	3½

(Sugar content estimated from values listed for carbohydrates in the various foodstuffs from: *Pennington JAT and Church HN: Bowes and Church's Food Values of Portions Commonly Used, 13th edition, 1980, Philadelphia, J. B. Lippincott Company.*)
Each teaspoon is equivalent to about 5 gm white granulated sugar.
Candy is generally composed of more than 75 percent sugar.

Starch ingestion interferes with iron absorption. Starch-induced anemia may involve alteration of the intestinal mucosa, causing a blockade of the iron absorption mechanism. It is also possible that iron binds to starch. Eating increased amounts of starch can be used as a protection against excessive iron absorption in susceptible persons. Dr. John Yudkin implicates sugar as a cause of obesity, diabetes, hyperinsulinism, high blood pressure, duodenal ulcers, fatty livers, atherosclerosis, certain forms of cancer, coronary and vascular disease, dental decay, gout, dermatitis, and a short lifespan.

Sugar irritates mucous membranes and stimulates the flow of gastric juice. Gallstones of cholesterol are common in people on refined diets, but almost unknown in primitive tribes. Similarly, appendicitis is almost unknown where refined foods are not eaten. The amount of sugar in a small candy bar is found naturally in about three pounds of apples.

Artificial sweeteners are not the answer to the sugar problem, as was widely believed a few years age. Cyclamates have been shown to produce a teratogenic (grossly deformed offspring) effect in rats if taken during the first two weeks of pregnancy. Infertility has also been reported, as have cancers. Saccharin appears to cause bladder tumors.

Ethanol (ordinary beverage alcohol) with the same number of calories as common table sugar (sucrose) produce fatty livers equally well. Pancreatitis often begins following a large meal, or following the ingestion of alcohol.

In Denmark during World War I, a severe drought and an Allied blockade caused massive starvation in 1917. Some 80% of the pigs and 66% of the cows were slaughtered for food. The need for livestock feed diminished. The cereals thereby saved were fed to the population in the form of whole rye bread with 12-15% wheat bran. The mortality from all causes fell in the first year by 17%, the lowest level ever seen in any country up to that time. When the great influenza pandemic struck in 1918, Denmark was the only country in Europe without an increase in mortality. The Danish death rate from all causes actually decreased, while in other European countries it rose by as much as 46%.

CHAPTER SIX

Fats

Chemical Composition of Fats

Fats (lipids) are substances, either liquid or solid, that are soluble in fat solvents. There are three types in the body: neutral fats (compounds of fatty acids with glycerin), phospholipids, and cholesterol. Fats have a negative charge on one end of the molecule and a positive charge at the other. On the positive end, there are hydrocarbons which are fat soluble. On the negative end, in the polar position, there is a water soluble part. The Divine Designer of chemicals devised this arrangement for the purpose of providing a useful tool in cellular physiology. By the direction of the turn of these chemicals, a membrane such as the cell wall can determine whether any given chemical will gain admission into the cell. By this means it can control the direction of the flow of chemicals, whether into or out of the cell.

Two other kinds of food lipids are cholesterol which occurs only in foods of animal origin, and phospholipids composed of phosphorus, fatty acids, glycerin, and nitrogenous compounds, the best known example being lecithin. We generally eat from 25-160 gm of fat per day. Fats are hard for the body to handle, a separate system of vessels having been designed to absorb and transport fats from the intestinal tract. Bile and pancreatic juices are required for lipid digestion. All fats are absorbed from the small intestine. About 60% of fats bypass the liver and are absorbed into the fluid of the lymphatic system (a much more slowly moving fluid than the blood) allowing for slower addition of the fats from the meal into the blood stream. The bile salts have a "detergent action" which results in an emulsion of the fats in the small intestine with the water available. Individual spherical particles are in the neighborhood of 500-1000 millimicra in diameter (a red blood cell is about 7000 millimicra).

These particles are further broken down by enzymes, which then form even smaller spheres with bile salts called micelles. The micelle is capable of being absorbed into the lymphatic vessel, as they have a diameter of only 5-10 millimicra. Short chain fats (less than 10 carbons) go directly into the blood stream. About 10% of the fat eaten is lost in the feces.

An interesting study was done using dogs fed high fat meals then forced to lie still by giving them a short acting anesthetic. After an hour the dogs woke up and began to move. At that time the dogs' arteries and capillaries were studied and found to contain large masses of fats which had accumulated during the period of inactivity following the meal. These masses can stop up the smaller capillaries, reducing the oxygen and nutrient delivery to the tissue cells. Also, fats in the blood serum alter the electrical charge on red blood cells, allowing them to clump together as shown in the illustration below.

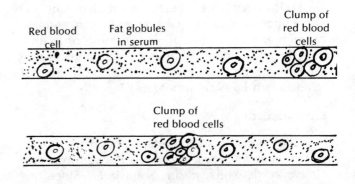

Two capillaries showing heavy fat content of serum, displacing other nutrients and causing clumping of red blood cells.

Triglycerides–Neutral Fats

Triglycerides occur in the body as adipose stores or as blood fats. Triglycerides may be taken into the body from foods or may be produced by the human body. A typical triglyceride is composed of a glycerine molecule and three fatty acids. Monoglycerides and diglycerides are also possible, that is, one glycerine molecule and one or two fatty acids.

Glycerol   Fatty Acid   Triglyceride

Phospholipids

Lecithin, a phospholipid, has only two fatty acids and a phosphate part. Crude lecithin, available commercially, causes a slight reduction in the cholesterol level of the blood. Purified lecithin does not possess this cholesterol-lowering property. It can be assumed that any benefit one might get from crude lecithin to lower blood cholesterol is from the other plant nutrients that accompany lecithin, and would, therefore, be present in the parent foods--grains, legumes, and seeds. It seems preferable to avoid taking lecithin, which would raise one's total lipid intake, and eat instead the whole foods from which lecithin is refined.

Lecithin contains a source of nitrogen (choline) and a phosphate group. Like oil, it is a concentrated nutrient and a form of fat. The free use of lecithin as a dietary supplement or as a therapeutic agent is unjustified and dangerous. It is a risk factor for atherosclerosis, as are other fats.[102]

Cholesterol

Cholesterol is an important physiologic sterol, classified as a lipid. The name is derived from two Greek words which mean "solid bile." Since bile occurs only in animal secretions, cholesterol will be found only in animal products. It is a natural component of every cell in the animal body, as it is present in the cell membrane. Cholesterol also forms a building block in the manufacture of certain steroidal hormones, such as those from the adrenal cortex and the sex glands. Any condition in

the life of a person that increases the need for extra hormones, such as the physical stress of illness or the various emotional stresses, will increase the production of cholesterol. Because cholesterol is so efficiently manufactured in the body, there is no daily requirement for it from any food.

Cholesterol

Cortisone

Testosterone

Progesterone

Estrogen
(Estradiol)

Physical and Chemical Properties of Fats

1. Insoluble in water.
2. Soluble in fat solvents.
3. Lighter weight than water (specific gravity 0.92-0.94 for fats as compared to 1.00 for water).
4. Capable of forming an emulsion with water. Examples of emulsions are mayonnaise and emulsified peanut butter. Finely divided droplets of water dispersed in fat form what is called an emulsion. Emulsions are more easily digested than unemulsified fats. Mayonnaise is approximately 80% fat in the commercial preparation, and 50% in the home-made variety.

5. Calorie content. Approximately nine calories per gram are furnished from fats. When we derive energy from palmitic acid, we get 41% efficiency in the metabolic systems. The animal body is an efficient machine. Steam and combustion engines don't do this well. Nevertheless, in our metabolic systems we derive only 3.69 calories per gram of fat at 41%. In the digestive tract, fats are emulsified with the aid of bile salts and are easily and almost completely broken up for absorption into the blood. Only about 10% of the fat eaten appears in the stool undigested.

Once an emulsion occurs, the fats are then in very tiny globules and are easily absorbed through the intestinal wall. Fat digestion begins in the stomach by gastric lipase. Fats are discharged from the stomach at a very regular rate of about ten grams per hour (about 2 teaspoons). When fat appears in the duodenum, a reflexive mechanism tells the stomach not to discharge more fat until that fat clears the duodenum. If a very large amount of fat is eaten, the hormone enterogastrone slows down stomach secretions and movement. This means that food may stay in the stomach for hours, promoting fermentation in the stomach with subsequent inflammation of the stomach lining (gastritis). The pylorus closes in response to the signal, and no more food leaves the stomach until the duodenum stops sending the message that fat is present. Then the pylorus will open up again and let more material out of the stomach which restarts the entire process. In the duodenum fat is more efficiently and completely digested by pancreatic lipase, a most powerful enzyme.

Once fats arrive in the bloodstream they are very difficult for the body to handle. For this reason fat absorption occurs in a different way from that of other nutrients. The blood vessels take up other nutrients directly into the blood stream. As mentioned earlier, over half the fats are taken up first into the lymphatics where they move slowly along, and over the course of several hours are gradually emptied into the left subclavian vein in the chest. Here, fats enter the blood stream. In this way, the body is protected from a great mass of fats that could prove fatal if absorbed directly into the blood stream. The body is protected by both the method of absorption and the slow emptying of fats from the stomach. Quigley described stomach evacuation in the following words: "A small portion of gastric contents enters the intestine. If the sample proves satisfactory, the remainder leaves the stomach rapidly; unsuitable material (that rich with fats, sugars, proteins, or certain other concentrated nutrients) initiates reactions from the duodenum which temporarily retard further gastric evacuation." (material in parenthesis not in quote)[103]

6. Saturation of fats. The carbons that make up a fat molecule have four electrical arms with which to attach other atoms. Two of the arms are used to attach the adjacent carbon atoms in the chain, and two are available to attach hydrogen atoms. If every available carbon arm is attached to hydrogen, the molecule is said to be saturated. If one arm refuses to attach to a hydrogen atom and doubles up with another electrical arm in an attachment to an adjacent carbon atom, the molecule is said to be unsaturated--monosaturated if only one carbon is involved in the doubling up of atoms, polyunsaturated if two or more carbons are involved. The hydrogenation of fats to make more carbon atoms in a chain carry two atoms of hydrogen is a chemical process which can be accomplished artificially to produce hard fats such as margarine; from soft or unsaturated fats of vegetable origin.

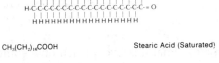

$CH_3(CH_2)_{16}COOH$ Stearic Acid (Saturated)

$CH_3(CH_2)_7CH=CH(CH_2)_7COOH$ Oleic Acid (Mono-unsaturated)

$CH_3(CH_2)_4CH=CHCH_2CH=CH(CH_2)_7COOH$ Linoleic Acid (Polyunsaturated)

$CH_3CH_2CH=CHCH_2CH=CH-CH_2-CH=CH(CH_2)_7COOH$ Linolenic Acid (Polyunsaturated)

18 Carbon Acids

The body cannot burn fatty acids with uneven numbers of carbon atoms, or very short chain fatty acids. The uneven saturated ones are often very irritating, as can be recognized from the following chart.

Chart of Fatty Acids

Length of Carbon Chain	Name of Fatty Acid	Where Found
2 carbon atoms	Acetic acid	Vinegar
4 carbon atoms	Butyric	Butter
6 carbon atoms	Caproic	Cheese
8 carbon atoms	Caprylic	Palm
10 carbon atoms	Capric	Goat wool
12 carbon atoms	Lauric	Milk, palm
14 carbon atoms	Myristic	Vegetables, nutmeg
16 carbon atoms	Palmitic	Palm, vegetables, milk

18 carbon atoms	Stearic	Animal fats
20 carbon atoms	Arachidic	Olives, peanuts
1 carbon atom	Formic	Ant and bee sting venom
3 carbon atoms	Propionic	Too low, irritant
5 carbon atoms	Valeric	Croton oil, cathartic
7 carbon atoms	Heptoic	Chemicals
9 carbon atoms	Nonylic	Chemicals
11 carbon atoms	Undecylic	Fungicides, (Athletes foot), industry
13 carbon atoms	Industrial chemicals	Industry
23 carbon atoms	Ecrucic	Mustard, pepper, etc.

When polyunsaturated fats are used in excess of the body's anti-oxidant controls, and the unsaturated fatty acid molecules break down to furnish free radicals, a chemical fragment is formed capable of combining with any available oxygen molecule to produce toxic peroxides. These are strong oxidizing agents that damage and destroy cells, leaving lipofuscin, a pigment found in aging cells.

7. The melting point. Oils are generally defined as fats which are liquid at room temperature. All vegetable oils are liquids, except coconut and chocolate fats which are solid at room temperature. Solid fats which congeal at room temperature, include all animal fats except fish oils, some of which are liquid.

Functions of Fats

Flavor. Most people agree that the addition of fat improves the flavor of food. However, there is a point at which adding more fat will not continue to improve the flavor, but will simply make it feel more greasy and add more calories. Usually a small fraction of the fat customarily added will be quite adequate to achieve the desired flavor enhancement. To add more fat simply produces a larger problem for the body to handle.

Satiety Value. The stomach containing fat slows its emptying, thereby causing it to fill earlier during the meal, and to remain filled longer after the meal has been taken. Some persons believe this slow emptying may prolong a sense of satiety and encourage the eating of smaller quantities. This point is not universally accepted; in fact, it may have the reverse effect in most people. It is known that fats promote fermentation in the stomach because of slow emptying. The irritation of the stomach, inflamed by the products of fermentation, causes it to be in motion more frequently, and to

be more likely to give a sensation of hunger, than is the healthy stomach which empties promptly without excessive fats.

All over America, frying is a favorite way to cook. Three times a day, the average American eats something fried. For breakfast he may get fried eggs, fried pancakes, fried toast (it may be oven fried), fried bacon or ham, fried potatoes, fried rice, or fried grits to name only a few. For dinner he may have fried hamburger, French fries, or a host of other things first fried and then smothered in gravy. Many feel that frying in liquid oil is better than frying in lard or saturated vegetable oil, but frying in any manner spoils the wholesomeness of the food.

What actually happens in frying? Temperatures up to 600-700 degrees F. may be obtained. At these temperatures *cis* fatty acids are converted to *trans* fatty acids. The difference between *cis* and *trans* is simply a matter of how the molecule is turned. This simple conversion, however, causes a reduction in the hypocholesteremic effect of unsaturated fatty acids. In other words, the unsaturated fats behave as if they were saturated. Thus, fried foods are more likely than unfried foods to increase the likelihood of developing hardening of the arteries.

When fat is reheated to frying temperatures the second time, as in a deep fat fryer, the fat is more likely to develop the cancer producing agent acrolein. Traces of benzopyrene have been found in fried foods. Significant quantities of this cancer-producing chemical are found in charcoal grilled meat. The fat from the meat drops onto the hot coals, is converted to benzopyrene, becomes a vapor in the heat, and redeposits on the steak. Benzopyrene is one of the most powerful carcinogens known.

Very hot temperatures destroy certain vitamins and may alter the major proteins. Most fried foods can be baked just as easily. Baking temperature is commonly 350 degrees F. for most recipes. Frying temperatures begin at 450 degrees and may reach 600-700 degrees during ordinary frying. If fried foods become burned or scorched, temperatures up to 1000 or 1100 degrees may have been reached.

The growth of malignant tumors in rats is stimulated by fats. This growth can be stimulated by either the subcutaneous injection of lard, or by feeding vegetable oil browned by heating. Another study shows that the feeding of heated polyunsaturated vegetable oil together with unheated vegetable oil increases the incidence of malignant tumors in rats exposed to a test cancer producing agent, 2-acetylaminofluorene.[104]

Fats and Heart Disease

The strong relationship between dietary fats and heart disease is now almost universally recognized. Literally thousands of studies have been published in the last three decades suggesting this relationship. Animal feeding experiments involving increased dietary fats and cholesterol almost always produce atherosclerosis, or fatty plaques, in blood vessels. Epidemiologic studies show the extremely high incidence of coronary heart disease in highly developed nations that consume large quantities of fat and cholesterol, and its virtual absence in developing countries where fat consumption is low. Other studies have shown that 45% of U. S. casualties in Viet Nam had evidence of significant coronary atherosclerosis, at an average age of 22.1 years! As many as 30% of sixth and seventh grade students already have abnormally high cholesterol levels (over 180 milligrams percent).[105]

Most of the early studies concentrated on cholesterol levels, with some consequent confusion occurring. While increasing levels of blood cholesterol seemed to be definitely correlated with increasing incidence of coronary heart disease when applied to an entire population group, it was not so nicely predictive when applied to the individual. The reasons for this apparent failure of correlations were several:

1. There has been an unfortunate tendency among researchers to equate *average* cholesterol levels with *normal* levels. Thus, nearly every U. S. laboratory lists 150-300 mg/dl as the "normal" for blood cholesterol. This range is widely accepted by most clinicians even today. The true "normal" blood cholesterol is not known. It is known that in nations of the world where coronary heart disease is virtually non-existent, blood cholesterol levels often average 100 mg/dl or less. We have practiced for years a convenient rule-of-thumb for the ideal blood cholesterol level of 100 plus the age. We feel we can confidently assure a person that he will never die of a heart attack if he maintains that level and a prudent lifestyle.

2. The recognition only in the past few years that one fraction of the total blood cholesterol, called "high density lipoprotein fraction" (HDL), is apparently protective against development of atherosclerosis. Thus, many people who have high total cholesterol levels are found to have high levels of the protective HDL cholesterol fraction, and do not develop vascular disease. HDL cholesterol levels are known to increase as a result of exercise

and stopping smoking.

3. The growing realization that not only saturated fats and cholesterol are involved, but the total fat intake is implicated, including polyunsaturated fats, which should also be severely limited by U. S. standards. This interesting finding was present in the report of earlier population studies, but was overlooked as being merely an indication of an impoverished diet. It remained for health promoters such as Nathan Pritikin to show that restriction of dietary fats of all kinds to 10% or less of total calories should be not only preventive, but apparently also curative of severe coronary heart disease. If Paul Dudley White or Michael deBakey had done the clinical experimental work that Pritikin has done, they would have received a Nobel Prize. But his work speaks for itself and is being confirmed daily in Health Conditioning Centers such as Yuchi Pines Institute, Wildwood, Spring Creek Ranch, Eden Valley, Living Springs, and others. (See Appendix for addresses) Some of our experience now spans a decade, standing the test of time.

4. The contribution of such prolonged and extensive studies as the Framingham study, which shows clearly that coronary heart disease is a lifestyle disease, multifactorial, and not related to only one or two factors.

The last chapter has not been written regarding fats, cholesterol, diet, and heart disease. But, we believe the evidence is clear that the very best diet to prevent coronary heart disease, or to treat it once developed, is one quite low (under 15%) in total fats; and preferably containing no animal fats, no exogenous cholesterol, and no refined sugar or grains; it would be relatively low in protein, and high in unrefined carbohydrates (fruits, vegetables, and whole grains).

Fat-Soluble Vitamins

Fats in foods carry the fat-soluble vitamins A, D, E, and K. Because these vitamins are more tenaciously held in the body by the fats than are the water soluble vitamins, one can more easily become overloaded on the fat-soluble vitamins. Therefore, toxicity to these vitamins represents the bulk of illnesses due to vitamin toxicities seen in the clinical practice of medicine.

Fatty Acid Content of Foods

Linoleic acid is a fatty acid the body cannot synthesize, and therefore, must acquire from food. Desaturation of other fats to form linoleic acid in the body cannot occur, as the desaturation process is not possible beyond carbon 9 in mammals. Since linoleic acid is an unsaturated 18 carbon fatty acid, it cannot be made by animals. It is found principally in fats of vegetable origin and has been considered to be protective to the heart, being capable of lessening the risk of high blood cholesterol or triglycerides.

Linoleic Acid
Two double bonds in this chain indicate
a polyunsaturated fatty acid.

If only 2% of the calories are in the form of linoleic acid, the body can get by. Corn oil is 50% linoleic acid. Many Chinese take only 3% of calories as fat, with no sign of fatty acid deficiency. Americans consume over 40% of their calories as fat. Linoleic acid is stored in adipose tissue, and it is unlikely that a deficiency would develop during moderate linoleic acid shortages, even when fairly prolonged.[106]

Mother's milk has more linoleic acid than does dairy milk. When taken in moderate quantities and in a diet not overbalanced with other fats, linoleic acid is a beneficial nutrient. If, however, linoleic acid is overused in the diet, especially if too many total fats comprise the diet, linoleic acid actually promotes the growth of cancer.[107] In this, we see illustrated that "more is not necessarily better," even of a good thing. The shorter fatty acids having 6, 8, or 10 carbons in the molecule are the part of butter fat which makes it soft. With sufficient time, linoleic acid placed in a container with water, will gradually become solid.

Sterols

Cholesterol is an animal product made by the liver for use in producing various hormones such as those from the ovaries and the adrenals. The liver can make cholesterol from almost any food, including plant sources yielding saturated fatty acids and acetate.

Plant oils are excellent sources of the plant steroid, phytosterol. Nuts and seeds contain moderate levels of plant sterols, and fruits and vegetables generally contain the lowest concentrations, with some exceptions. Phytosterols are composed of 28 or 29 carbon sterols, whereas cholesterol is a 27 carbon sterol. An increased phyto-

sterol intake is associated with a lowering of the blood cholesterol and may actually decrease the intestinal absorption of both dietary cholesterol and that formed by the liver and excreted in bile.

Cholesterol

Ergosterol
(plant sterol)

7-Dehydrocholesterol
(in skin a pro-vitamin D)

7-Dehydrocholesterol occurs in the skin and is converted to a vitamin D upon irradiation with ultraviolet. Irradiation of ergosterol also yields a Vitamin D. Ergosterol is produced by plants. Each of these sterols is called a "pro-vitamin D." Note their similiarity to cholesterol.

Nine different phytosterols are identified in plant oils. Refining of oils causes the oil to contain 20-60% less total sterol than the crude oils as found in the plant or fruit. Hydrogenation further reduces the sterol content from 20-40% beyond that of the refining processes. However, in olive oil, most of the major sterols may be stabilized by prolonged heating at 180 degrees Centigrade.

Some rough guidelines as to the amounts of plant sterols in specific foodstuffs are obtained from studies being done in Japan. The following shows the foods highest in plant sterols in each of the several groups:[108]

Oils	mg./100 gm.
Chestnut oil	5,350
Rice bran oil (crude)	3,225
Sesame seed oil	2,950
Spinach seed oil	1,827
Rye germ oil	2,425
Alfalfa seed oil	2,080
Wheat germ oil	1,970
Corn oil	1,390
Sunflower oil	725
Mustard seed oil	624
Pumpkin seed oil	523
Rape seed oil (crude)	513
Peanut oil (crude)	337

(Young mung beans have more sterol than older tissues.)

Vegetables	Mg/100 gm (fresh weight)
Dry barley seedlings	234
Common bean seedlings	121
Beets	25
Brussell sprouts	24
Corn (depends on strain)	60-70
Oriental pickling melon	28
Okra	24
Pea seedlings	108
Radish greens	34
Immature soybeans	50
Dry vetch	52

Fruits	mg./100gm. (edible portion of fruit)
Figs	31
Lemon peelings	35
Pomegranate	17
Strawberry	12

Seeds and Nuts	mg./100 gm.
Sesame seeds	714
Sunflower seeds	534

Spices	mg./100 gm
Sage	244
Oregano	203

Cereals	mg./100 gm.
Rice bran	1325

For Durum and hard red spring wheat, the sterol content is highest in the bran, in soft wheats, highest in the head shorts.

Legumes	mg./100 gm. (edible portion)
Peanuts	220
Soybeans	161
Peanut butter	102

Plant sterols are found in generous quantity in the following foods:

Fruits	Legumes
Apples	Calabar beans
Cherries	Peanuts
Olives	Soy products
Plums	

Tubers	Nightshades
Carrots	Eggplant
Yams	Tomatoes
	Potatoes
	Peppers

Herbs	Grains
Alfalfa	Cereal grains except rye, buck-wheat, and white rice
Anise seed	
Garlic	
Licorice root	
Parsley	**Others**
Red raspberry	Coconut
Sage	Food yeast
Oregano	Wheat germ

Bile Salts and Bile Acids

These substances are necessary for the absorption of cholesterol and other lipids from the small intestines. Fiber tends to attach to the bile salts and acids, thereby making cholesterol absorption difficult. The whole group of chemicals, fiber, cholesterol, and bile products go out together in the fecal stream. Several studies have shown that certain vegetable fibers and gums such as in rolled oats, Bengal gram, guar gum, and pectin are more efficient in lowering cholesterol than are wheat fiber, cellulose, and lignin. The reasons for and implications of the observations are not completely clear at this time.

Fats Related to Sugar

A rat or human may be "primed" with generous quantities of sucrose in the diet. If radiocarbon labled sucrose is then given, more radiocarbon will be found in fat stores. When a glucose tolerance test is done using sucrose, more radiocarbon is incorporated into the fat than if the glucose tolerance test uses glucose. This will cause a more rapid synthesis of fat. Sucrose causes an increase of triglycerides by its deleterious effect on insulin. Fructose does not stimulate the release of insulin to the degree that glucose does. Therefore, fructose in usual dosages does not stimulate the pancreas to produce insulin as well as does glucose. Starch, which breaks down into glucose, stimulates the pancreas more strongly than fruits containing fructose.

The clearance of fat from the blood after a meal is not as efficient if one has taken sucrose (common table sugar) in the meal than if no free sugar is used. This may be demonstrated by giving a load of 60 grams of fat and 25 grams of sucrose at breakfast. Then the level of insulin is measured. The insulin levels in the blood after a meal are not as high with sucrose as with glucose, since sucrose is half fructose, which does not stimulate the pancreas to produce insulin as strongly as glucose. If the blood levels of cholesterol and triglycerides are measured at the same time as insulin, these values will be higher with sucrose than with glucose, since insulin helps clear the blood of fats. Fructose in the diet, whether from sucrose or from fruits, allows the fat to stay in the blood longer than does glucose. To summarize, we can say that studies show that sweets generally cause much more harm in the body when eaten with fats than either nutrient causes when taken alone.

CHAPTER SEVEN

Proteins

Composition of Proteins

Proteins are composed of large molecules made up of a number of simpler units called amino acids. Amino acids contain nitrogen in each molecule. These basic units contain at least one organic acid radical (-COOH) and one amino group (-NH₂). Some amino acids contain two of one group or the other, and one amino acid (cystine) contains two of each. There are 23 different amino acids which are known to be present in nature and are available for use in

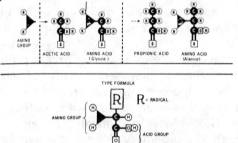

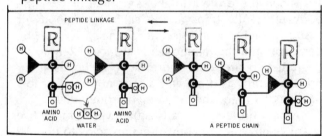

-NH₂: Amine radical. -COOH: Organic acid radical. -R: Remainder of molecule.

the formation of proteins. The number of different amino acid molecules which comprise the various proteins of the body varies from eight to eighteen.

After absorption of the amino acids from the gastrointestinal tract and inspection by the liver, the blood carries the amino acids to the tissues where selection is made for formation of individual proteins to be used in various body processes, even for thinking. Eight of the 23 amino acids cannot be manufactured from other substances in sufficient quantity in the animal body and are said to be essential; that is, these amino acids must be supplied in the diet of man and animals from plants. The essential amino acids are: isoleucine, leucine, lysine, methionine, phenylalanine, threonine, tryptophan, and valine. All animals require these amino acids from an outside source. They are originally synthesized by plants, and it seems reasonable for man to obtain them from the original source as do most animals.

Organic acids, such as amino acids, are defined as chemical compounds that have a carboxylic acid group (a carbon with two oxygen atoms and a hydrogen atom grouped together and designed as a -COOH group) on their molecules. In addition to the specific chemical arrangements of atoms, there are physical characteristics of proteins and other chemical compounds that assist in classification of all organic chemicals. Organic chemicals are carbon compounds produced by living organisms. Fats and carbohydrates are relatively small, simple molecules, whereas, proteins are large and complex. The fats and carbohydrates contain carbon, hydrogen, and oxygen. Proteins contain nitrogen in addition to these basic atoms. Most proteins also contain sulfur. Many contain phosphorus and iron as well. They are formed by joining amino acids together in a special type of chain linkage called "peptide linkage."

Proteins are present in all living tissue. There are certain specialized proteins such as nucleoproteins and hemoglobin. There is a limitless variety of proteins possible from the 23 amino acids that are present in nature. The proteins differ in the way the amino acids are joined together allowing them to form different geometric configurations. They may be round, long, woven, intermeshed, quilted, etc. The round ones, or globular proteins, have a distinct function based partly on roundness. The globin part of the hemoglobin name comes from a globular protein. The fibrillar ones are long strings of carbon compounds which do not fold or bend upon themselves, but stretch out in long groups. They, too, have distinct functions based partly on being stringy. Fibrin, the tangled meshwork of blood clot and fibrous connective tissue that holds the various body parts together, are examples of the fibrillar variety.

From Bogert, Briggs and Calloway. NUTRITION & PHYSICAL FITNESS, 9th ed. W.B. Saunders Co., 1973.

A peptide linkage joins the amino acids in all proteins. The peptide linkage is broken by digestion before proteins can be absorbed into the blood stream. The type of digestion that breaks peptide linkages is spoken of as peptic digestion, done by pepsin, a digestive enzyme of the stomach. Many believe proteins to be the most important of the nutrients, not because they need to be present in the greatest quantity in the diet, but because protein deprivation results in such serious disturbances in the function of the body. In protein deficiency, there may be inhibition of growth, reduction of mental capacity, and a reduced sense of well-being.

Protein Absorbed More Efficiently in Shortages

When the protein intake is normal or low, the body efficiently traps amino acids from food for tissue protein synthesis. In animals, it can be demonstrated that amino acids are less likely to be degraded to urea and more likely to be used for protein synthesis if animals are on a normal or low protein diet than when on a high protein diet.

A high protein diet causes the liver to make five adaptive enzymes to convert amino acids to urea.[109] The liver relaxes its efforts as the intake of protein goes down. Adaptive mechanisms are quite active to increase trapping and recycling of protein when no excess exists.[110] The adaptive responses seen in liver enzymes reflect the composition of the metabolic status with accuracy.[111] To degrade protein to urea and excrete it in the urine is wasteful, both of food and of metabolic energy. Nibbling as compared with eating meals leads to poorer absorptive capacity of the digestive tract,[112] and presumably less availability of protein. It can be readily understood that it is advantageous from an economic standpoint, and to relieve the digestive and urinary tracts, to have a regular meal pattern with nothing between meals in order to obtain the most efficient utilization of foods in the gastrointestinal tract.[113]

Are We Eating Too Much Protein?

An excess of protein in the American diet probably decreases lifespan, and an excess produces no known benefit. There is no possibility of increasing muscle mass by eating extra protein, yet athletes eat enormous amounts of high protein foods on the mistaken advice of colleagues or coaches that muscle development will be better with extra protein. The usual athlete takes in three to five times the recommended daily allowance. Further, the average sedentary American eats at least twice as much protein as is needed. The National Research Council has been gradually reducing its recommended daily allowance from one gm/kg of body weight to 0.9 gm/kg, to 0.8 gm/kg. Levels as low as 0.2 gm/kg have been used effectively for long-term maintenance of patients with kidney disease. This means that an average 150 pound man would need only 14 grams of protein each day, the amount found in 4 slices of bread, or 5/8 cup of lima beans, or 1½ cups of split pea soup, or 1½ cups of Brussells sprouts.

Animal evidence used against excess protein for humans includes increased activity of enzymes associated with protein and amino acid metabolism, and increased urea formation with feeding excess protein. The kidneys of animals enlarge on long-term high protein diets due to the excess work load. Albumin and casts increase in animal urine. Rabbits on high protein diets develop nephritis. Trout fed a low protein diet live twice as long as trout fed a high protein diet. Humans are affected in much the same way as animals on a high protein diet according to studies at Mayo Medical School. A low protein, low liquid diet has been used for patients with chronic renal disease with much promise. The need for dialysis can be postponed in some patients, and the frequency of dialysis can be reduced in those already being dialyzed. Dr. Ralph A. Nelson describes increased protein intake as idling our metabolic engine at a faster rate.

In metabolizing protein in the body, ammonia can be formed as a by-product. This ammonia is usually of low concentration in the body, which is fortunate, as it is a toxic waste. Intestinal absorption of ammonia occurs chiefly in the colon, and comes from the following sources: (1) that formed from urea by bacterial ureases; (2) that present in amides formed as products of protein digestion; (3) that coming from medications. Renal formation of ammonia is from glutamine. Muscle formation of ammonia occurs during exercise.

The best advice scientists can offer after half a century of nutrition research, is to eat a well-balanced diet, not a high protein diet. Recent research by Willard J. Visek of Cornell University supports this view. When people eat too much protein or have an unbalanced diet, harmful amounts of ammonia may be released. Cell culture experiments show that ammonia slows the growth of normal cells more than that of cancer cells. Ammonia changes the character of RNA, the cell's regulator of protein manufacture. It also alters the rate at which thymidine is used for DNA, the cell's genetic material. These are features of protein metabolism which make cells less able to protect themselves from infection and from malignant transformation. The unanswered question of these findings, however, is the one underlying the bulk of medical research: Do cells inside the human body act the same way they do in tissue cultures in the laboratory? In this case, Visek believes they do. Cells in the body are exposed to ammonia every time protein is digested. The more protein the greater the likelihood of producing damaging quantities of ammonia.[114]

Weight loss diets high in protein and low in carbohydrate, cause adverse side reactions that include breakdown of some protein tissues and increased urinary excretion of calcium and other minerals, according to a study reported by Harold Yacowitz, Ph.D of the Health Research Institute at Fairleigh Dickinson University, Madison, New Jersey. "The increased calcium excretion may be the result of some loss of bone matrix," he told the 57th annual meeting of the Federation of American Societies for Experimental Biology. To determine the biochemical changes in the blood and urine of people following widely used crash diets of the Stillman variety, Dr. Yacowitz studied five overweight but otherwise healthy men and women. They were allowed free choice of their regular diets for two weeks, followed by one or two weeks on the high protein, low-carbohydrate diet. During both periods, each subject received a vitamin-mineral capsule daily. All subjects on the high-protein diet lost between five and nine pounds, but there was significant increase in the level of serum glutamic oxalacetic transaminase (SGOT) indicative of protein tissue breakdown. There were also significant increases in urinary excretion of calcium, phosphorus, iron, and zinc during the high-protein test period. Magnesium excretion also increased, but not significantly. Based on these high urinary mineral excretion levels, along with similar data on

calcium excretion reported by other research workers, it appears that loss of bone matrix occurs on a high-protein diet. This was Dr. Yacowitz's conclusion from the study.[115]

There are 380-400 thousand hemoglobin molecules in one red blood cell. Two million red blood cells are being produced in the body every minute. This requires an enormous turnover of protein. Fortunately the body is very efficient in conserving its building material, and much of the protein is reused again and again.

Even though the non-essential amino acids can be produced in the body, these amino acids are made so slowly that we could never keep up with our needs. Therefore, we must think in terms of getting *all* the essential and *most* of the non-essential amino acids from the diet. The terms "essential" and "non-essential" in referring to amino acids are unfortunate and have contributed greatly to our misunderstanding of protein. If we get a wide variety of unrefined foods, concentrating on fruits and vegetables, getting plenty of grains, and occasionally a few nuts, we can be certain we are getting all the nutrients the Creator intended.

Although the brain weighs only 2% of the total body weight, it uses a maximum of 25% of the body's total energy. Nutrition of brain and nerve cells is different from nutrition of the other cells. There is the so-called "blood-brain barrier" which holds back from the brain tissue the higher concentrations of many of the nutrients, particularly amino acids, to which other cells and tissues have free access. This mechanism attempts to protect the brain from damaging effects of over concentration of nutrients in the blood. It can be easily overpowered.

Many of the detoxifying processes of the liver make use of sulfur, a fact which may have some relation to the liver's protecting action of the sulfur containing amino acids. The accumulation of toxins to the abnormal concentrations of waste products resulting from a liver injury may cause damage to cerebral tissue directly. As a result of such irritants, there develops an increased number of protoplasmic astrocytes in the cortex, brain nuclei, thalamus, pons, etc. Astrocytes (star shaped cells) are not part of the functioning apparatus of the brain, but of the connective tissue support. An increase in this tissue can crowd the nerve cells. How important to protect every function of the body so that the precious brain can be preserved with all its priceless functions throughout a long lifetime!

Naming Errors in Nutrition

There are several naming errors in nutrition that are gradually being corrected. One of these naming errors that has led to misunderstanding and a wrong emphasis is that of "complete" and "incomplete" proteins. So-called "complete proteins" are defined as those that supply all the essential amino acids in proper balance and amounts needed for the formation of human tissue protein. A dietary containing such a balance is said to be of high biologic value. If there are certain essential amino acids in low supply, the protein is said to be "incomplete," or of lower biologic value.

Actually, the use of the terms, complete and incomplete proteins, is misleading, because all natural foods contain all of the essential amino acids, and no food protein is so perfect as to be the total answer to all our protein needs.[116] A better way to speak of proteins is that of high or low biologic value. Not all nuts contain high quality proteins. Therefore, a wide variety of foods in the diet makes up for the deficiencies of a single food by mutual supplementation.

Legumes represent an increasingly important place in the American diet, particularly as population increases and food stores decrease. Since 2800 B. C. soybeans have rated a place with the five principal crops in China: rice, wheat, barley, millet, and soybeans. Soybeans are very versatile, and in addition to being eaten plain, may be made into pastas, cheeses, loaves, sauces, and curds. When used along with a staple diet of cereals, they furnish a well-balanced array of amino acids. Legumes are abundant in lysine but deficient in methionine. When grains are also present in the dietary, this deficiency is readily supplied. Soybeans contain more protein than any other commonly used legume. When using dry beans (legumes) as a main dish, an individual serving should amount to about 250-325 calories. However, the portions should be only about 100 calories when used as a vegetable, because of the concentration of nutrients and the difficulty experienced by some persons to digest a lot of heavy food. Beans may be eaten by most people at any meal if not eaten in large quantity, just as nuts.

There is an amino acid pool[117] from which amino acids are drawn to produce proteins and other compounds, From this source, amino acids are pulled for energy needs. When the intake and output of amino acids in this pool are approximately balanced, a person is said to be in nitrogen or protein equilibrium. If one is in "positive nitrogen balance," the intake is greater than output. A "negative balance" indicates that the output is greater than the intake. An excess of certain amino acids may reduce or in some instances, increase the absorption of another amino acid.

For optimum protein synthesis and most efficient utilization of amino acids, it is desirable to have all of the amino acids present in the gastrointestinal tract and available to the various tissues at the same time. In times of privation or restricted variety of foods the balance of amino acids can be provided from the amino acid pool for a short time. Eventually, it is necessary to restock the amino acid pool with a wider variety of amino acids than can be derived from a diet of all nuts or all cereals or all fruits. For this reason, the Master Designer built into our brains an appetite for a variety of foods, and supplied the world with an endless array of produce to satisfy the appetite for variety. In this way, all of the amino acids can be supplied in sufficient quantity and proportion to provide for adequate protein synthesis.

The average person should not have the slightest concern when approaching meals as to whether or not all of the amino acids may be present in the diet. One should eat with thanksgiving and not be afraid of becoming deficient. The time to do careful planning is at the time policies are set in the household, menus are fashioned, food is purchased, or gardens planted. Then the matter should be banished from the thoughts and no anxiety developed over it. If you think your food will hurt you, be assured that it will.

Uses of Protein in the Body

Protein is not utilized for energy in muscular work if calories are adequate from carbohydrates. This is spoken of as the "protein sparing" action of carbohydrates. Perhaps the ideal in nutrient intake is that about 70-80% of the caloric requirements be furnished by complex carbohydrates. In other countries, the intake may be somewhat different because of food traditions and marketing supplies. The Chinese diet in some areas resembles the following percentages:

Cereals and legumes	88%
Vegetables and fruits	5%
Fats	4%
Meat, eggs, and milk	3%

Since almost 100% of carbohydrates can be converted to energy, they are most efficiently used in metabolism and are the least expensive forms of fuel. Carbohydrates have the smallest amount of residue left over for the body to dispose of, or to accumulate as wastes. Protein is an expensive fuel, "burns" inefficiently (only 58%), and has much waste left over for detoxification and excretion.

New tissue. Skin, hair, scars, mucosa of the gastrointestinal tract, formation of new blood, and repair of injured cells in such organs as liver and pancreas all require protein. The lining of the gastrointestinal tract is one of the most active tissues in the body, being entirely renewed every one and one-half days. If there is any interference in protein synthesis, the gastrointestinal tract will soon reflect this fact by a sore tongue, abdominal pain, diarrhea, gastrointestinal bleeding, or other symptoms.

Precursor elements. *Cell maturation* is dependent on certain substances that come from protein, and without them, maturation of cells cannot occur. *Enzymes* are enormously useful in numerous functions of the body. Their formation is dependent on proteins. *Hormones* have certain portions that come from proteins as a part of the skeleton of each molecule. Examples are the *thyroid hormone* which contains the amino acid tyrosine, and serotinin, a hormone produced in the intestinal tract and in portions of the central nervous system, which contains the amino acid metabolyte tryptamine. *Antibodies* are produced in response to a stimulus from a foreign substance which the body considers a threat. The antibodies are fashioned from amino acids by lymphocytes. They represent one of our first lines of defense against germ invasion and allergenic substances. At least one B-vitamin, *niacin,* has a large part in its skeleton made up by the amino acid tryptophane. Other vitamins have their metabolism greatly influenced by proteins. *Hemoglobin* and *myoglobin* may both be inadequately formed if there is insufficient protein to form the globin parts of their molecules.

Regulation. The hemoglobin buffer system is an example of an important mechanism for maintenance of acid-base balance which depends on adequate protein. Because of osmotic pressure built up by proteins in the blood, the excessive build up of tissue fluid is prevented. One improper effect of a high protein diet is that excessive quantities of water are removed from the tissues by the osmotic pull of proteins and their waste products in the blood. Water and electrolyte balance are thereby threatened.

Upkeep. During times of emotional or physical stress, and during the most active periods of muscular activity and reproduction, there is a need for more protein than in old age. Since hormones are needed in stress, both fats and proteins may be used more in general metabolism in periods of stress. Also, in the healing of burns, replacing blood following hemorrhage, and in many other stressful conditions, there needs to be an especially well balanced supply of proteins. Care should be exercised, however, not to take in a great excess of protein, as the imbalance places a special strain on the metabolic systems.

Choline is a detoxifier, assists in the transport of fats, assists in nerve transmission, and can compensate for shortages in other amino acids, such as methionine. Choline-high foods may be given to good advantage in nervous disorders, overweight, and infections such as streptococcal sore throat. Choline is necessary for the synthesis of the serum phospholipid which forms an active component of the inhibitor of the hemolysin made by streptocci called streptolysin S. Choline may have protective principles that guard against rheumatic fever.[118] Good sources of choline are yeast, legumes (soybeans, peanuts, beans, and peas), and wheat germ.

Plant proteins give a reduction in serum cholesterol levels, whereas animal protein causes an elevation of serum cholesterol.

Milk production. Among the activities requiring a more generous supply of protein is that of lactation. The pregnant or nursing mother should have her food needs generously supplied.

Energy. If calories from fats and carbohydrates are inadequate, proteins will be used to supply energy. Since proteins are generally more expensive than other foods that supply calories, to use a diet high in protein is poor economy.

Daily Requirements of Protein

The average adult needs less than 30 grams of protein per day. All unrefined foods contain protein. Fruit contains 1-3 grams and vegetables 2-8 grams per serving. Bread furnishes 3.5-4 grams per slice, 1 cup of steamed soybean sprouts furnishes 15 grams as do 1¾ cups of collards, 2 cups of broccoli, 1 cup of peas, and a few walnuts. On a natural diet, if one takes care of the calories, the protein will take care of itself.

Men and women can live without apparent harm on protein intakes of 25-40 grams from vegetable foods. In 1964, Rose said that a daily intake of eighteen grams of protein, carefully selected, would probably be sufficient. In 1971, Hegsted reduced the figure to approximately ten grams, because the body is so efficient in recycling amino acids.

Such a heavy emphasis has been given to proteins in this country, that many people are worried about getting enough, when most are actually consuming toxic quantities. A balance of body chemicals is needed, rather than a surplus of any one. All nutrients, including water and oxygen, produce toxic symptoms when taken into the body in too great a quantity.

The most abundant chemical in the body is water. The second most abundant chemical is protein. The animal cell membrane is approximately 60% protein and 40% lipids. About 10-20% of the cellular content is protein; 2-3% is lipid. Carbohydrates, usually in the form of glycogen, comprise approximately one percent of the substance of cells. Glycogen is a polymer of glucose. That is, it is composed of multiple units of glucose joined together.

Nutritive Effect of Foods Near to Pharmacologic Effects

To many it is a new idea that there are naturally occurring substances in foods that affect physiologic processes in measurable ways, both beneficially and adversely; making it possible to alter the function of the body through diet. Toxicities from foods are known to involve the nervous system (psychologic and neurologic), immune system, cardiovascular system, skin, urinary tract, the unborn child, and many other systems, organs, and tissues. Not only acute poisonings, such as mushroom poisoning, but chronic long-term disease may be produced by food ingredients. Some of the substances occurring in foods cause behavioral and social alterations, at times of major proportions.[119]

Chemical compounds that adversely affect us may be encountered in naturally occurring substances such as solanine in potatoes, which may cause acute toxicity at times and arthritis on a chronic basis in some individuals. A second effect is through contaminants such as aflatoxins, which can cause cancer, in improperly stored peanuts. A third way that toxic effects of food chemicals cause chronic disease is from genetic abnormalities causing enzyme deficiencies, --well known examples being phenylketonuria, lactose intolerance, and favism. The number of the enzyme deficiency states is rapidly rising, and may themselves be produced by toxic substances in foods, notably caffeine. A fourth factor relevant to food chemical

toxicity is the interaction between food components and those of the host, or interactions between foods when several foods are eaten at once. An illustration of the reactions is the union of nitrates and nitrites with amines to form nitrosamines; very potent cancer producers.

Some of the beneficial effects of foods used in disease states are given elsewhere, as in the endocrinology section. To avoid the harmful effects, a good policy is that of preparing foods by cooking according to the best possible practices, selecting foods known to be safe by long use in population groups, and keeping the number of dishes served at a meal to two or three with bread.

Types of Protein

There are many different types of proteins, some superior to others and some being quite efficient in their ability to supply the body's needs. Still fresh in the mind are the sudden deaths that occurred from the high protein diets given for weight control. The protein was of such an inferior quality that it could not support life. Those who were the most faithful on the diet and stuck to it the longest suffered worse. This tragedy illustrates vividly the necessity to be reasonable in diet and to adhere to what is being or has been done by large population groups for hundreds or thousands of years, rather than shifting to fads or drifting with the careless.

Simple proteins include albumins, globulins, glutelins, prolamins, albuminoids, histones, and protamines. Conjugated proteins include nucleoproteins, mucoproteins, glycoproteins, lipoproteins, phosphoproteins, chromoproteins, and metalloproteins. Derived proteins are products formed in the various stages of hydrolysis, such as proteoses, peptones, polypeptides, and peptides. Digestion produces many derived proteins which act as toxins in the body.

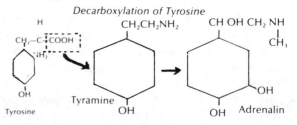

Decarboxylation of Tyrosine

Amino acids generally are not very active pharmacologically. But upon removal of the carboxyl acid group (COOH), inert amino acids are transformed into highly active amines as illustrated above. Tyrosine becomes tyramine which is a near relative of adrenalin.

Both tyramine and adrenalin raise blood pressure and have other profound influences on the body. Tyramine is not only produced in the colon, but is found in cheese. Tryptamine from tyramine also raises blood pressure.

The action of intestinal bacteria on amino acids produces some derived proteins and other substances such as phenol, cresol, indole, and skatole. These are transported to the liver and conjugated with sulfuric acid, forming sulfates which are less toxic than their precursors.

Some Decomposition Products of Amino Acids in the Colon

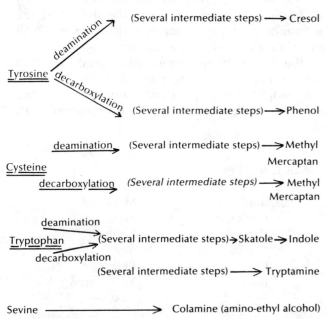

The amino acids are listed on the left. All of the end products found on the right in the above equations are harmful to a greater or lesser degree. Cresol and phenol are irritants. Methyl mercaptan has a marked blood pressure lowering effect. Skatole and indole give a foul odor to the stool, and when given in large quantities by mouth can produce headache and dizziness. Tryptamine can raise blood pressure, and Colamine is toxic in the same way as alcohol.

Simple proteins are those that yield only amino acids on hydrolysis. In the body and in foods, simple proteins are predominant. Albumins which are simple proteins, are readily soluble in water and are those that are chiefly present in animal fluids. Albumin is a small, fibrillar shaped molecule. If there is damage to the small tubules of the kidney, albumin can readily leak out, as it is a slender molecule. Therefore, albumin is the protein most commonly found in the urine during a diseased state. Less readily soluble proteins are those that are found in grains, such as gluten in wheat and zein in corn. Regardless of the source of protein, the blood protein level is maintained in a very constant and consistent level and pattern, unless serious metabolic, nutritional, or disease states occur.

Conjugated proteins are more complex and are comprised of amino acids and some non-protein substance such as fats (lipoproteins) or carbohydrates (glycoproteins). Lipoproteins are found in blood, and glycoproteins are found in mucus. Hemoglobin is bound to an iron portion, and nucleoproteins are bound to necleic acid.

Deoxyribonucleic acid (DNA), a nucleoprotein, is present in all cell nuclei, but differs slightly from individual to individual and more markedly from species to species. These substances contain nitrogenous bases and have a code that arranges the various genetic specifications of each individual. Only four nitrogenous bases are found in DNA: adenine, guanine, thymine, and cytosine. The code is rearranged for such matters as sending messages from one cell to another or from one part of the same cell to another.

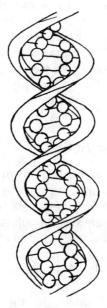

In 1935, about 56% of the protein from food in the American diet was of animal origin. Since then the percentage has jumped to 68%. It is difficult to devise a diet with a higher percentage of protein than approximately 15% of the total calories unless purified or refined proteins are added. Since most foods contain only 16-30% of their weight as actual proteins, the rest being present as fat, water, and carbohydrates, a higher protein percentage could be accomplished only by the addition of purified proteins. This natural feature of foods goes far to help prevent injury from toxic overload of proteins.

Most Americans have been educated to believe they will become dificient in amino acids if they do not eat animal proteins. The fallacy of such an idea is clearly illustrated by a consideration of the analysis of ordinary white wheat flour. White flour has as much or more of the essential amino acids (other than lysine) than either whole egg or beef muscle. Of course, whole wheat would be even better. Lysine, the amino acid low in grains, is easily supplied from greens or legumes.

Because of the presence of the amino acid pool, there is a dynamic equilibrium between the proteins in the cells and the amino acids resulting from digestion of protein in the foods. Absorption of dietary amino acids is facilitated by secretion of a spread of amino acids from the body's protein pool. Amino acids slip back and forth as needed; therefore, the emphasis given by some to obtain a completely balanced protein with each meal is not well placed, as the natural selection of the appetite will easily accomplish the matter. The serious problem arises in the use of "empty calories," derived from food essentially devoid of any nutrients other than those that produce energy. In the United States, empty calories represent 30% of the total calories, or 1,175 calories per day. If we add refined cereals instead of whole grain cereals such as oatmeal, we add 17% more empty calories, which is almost half of the total calories consumed by most Americans.

Specific Dynamic Action

The specific dynamic action of food is the stimulus given to the metabolism, mainly by proteins, but to a lesser degree by carbohydrates and fats. A high protein diet stimulates metabolism. This stimulus acts as a tax, not a relief, to the body. Osmotic relationships, antibodies, and plasma globulins are all related to a proper intake of proteins.

There is no advantage to the individual in eating a high protein diet in anticipation of some future need. The time for using extra protein in the diet is during or immediately after the time of the stress or period of privation, not before. The amount of work or exercise one does is not of prime importance in determining protein allowances. An office worker needs about as much protein as a logger in the cold, north woods.

There is a sense of well-being initially observed from a high protein intake which comes from the stimulus to the metabolism, related to the heat of specific dynamic action. On the other hand, many who begin a vegetarian diet mistakenly feel that they are low in protein if they experience a sensation of weakness. While the stimulatory effect is lost, by testing there is no actual reduction in muscular strength or endurance, only a sensation of weakness. The sensation lessens in about five days. A genuine protein deficiency is accompanied by edema, retardation of growth, wasting of body tissues, true muscle weakness, and loss of vigor.

Purine Content of Foods

The use of a high protein diet adds to the burden of elimination of the kidneys, the liver, and the gastrointestinal tract. Another toxic effect of a high protein diet is the gradual accumulation of purines in the blood. Purine degradation produces such waste products as uric acid. Elevated uric acid levels are associated with gout and kidney stones. They also may represent a risk factor for coronary heart disease.

Group 1: High Purines

Anchovies	Mussels
Bouillon	Mackerel
Goose	Sardines
Gravy	Scallops
Organ meats	Roe
Pork	Partridge
Beef	Yeast (brewer's and baker's)

Group 2: Moderate Purines

All other meats and fish	Asparagus
Brains	Mushrooms
Poultry	Spinach
Shellfish	Lentils
Dry beans	

Group 3: Negligible

Whole grain bread and cereals	Rice
Fruits	Vegetables (other than those listed above)
Nuts	
Olives	Avocado
	Corn bread
	Popcorn

Disease caused by pure protein deficiency is probably unknown. It was once thought that kwashiorkor was a pure protein deficiency. It has been determined that providing these children with balanced amino acids in the absence of making up their needed calories, vitamins, fatty acids, and minerals will fail to cure kwashiorkor. The accepted terminology now is "protein-calorie deprivation," and the syndrome requires the additional factor of acute or chronic infection, diarrhea, or parasitism.

Brain Proteins

Five brain proteins in the form of enkephalins are reported to be natural pain killers. The enkephalins are a part of a 31 amino acid protein called beta-endorphins, which are themselves a part of a 91 amino acid protein called beta-lipotropin. These proteins are produced in the brain, and apparently do a variety of things: relieve pain, improve learning, reduce memory loss, induce pleasure, and induce seizures.[122] Regularly, there are new chemicals discovered in the brain that give the student of neurophysiology a glimpse of the great genius of the Creator. Let us be thankful for the opportunity to learn of His handiwork.

CHAPTER EIGHT

Vitamins

The Vital Amines

The "vital amines" were discovered at about the turn of our century. Since some were soon found not to be amines, the word "vitamin" (dropping the "e") was coined in 1912. They are considered to be "biologic catalysts." Vitamins are defined as carbon compounds that cannot be synthesized by our own bodies and are needed only in minute quantities. They became known because of the deficiency diseases that resulted from their absence in the diet. Replacement of the vitamins results in a dramatic relief of symptoms in most cases. Many co-enzymes essential to specific body functions are partly vitamins. While vitamins are not synthesized by the body, some including vitamins K, B-1, folacin, and B-12 are synthesized by bacteria in various parts of the body. All of these are produced by microorganisms that normally inhabit the gastrointestinal tract. Vitamin B-12 is also produced in the mouth, conjunctival sacs, tonsils, nasopharynx, bronchial tree, sinuses, stomach, and small bowel.

Twenty vitamins are known to be important in human nutrition. The vitamins fall naturally into two groups: fat soluble (A, D, E, and K), and water soluble vitamins (B complex and C). The water soluble vitamins are fairly easily excreted in case of excessive intake, even though it is an energy using process to absorb them through the small intestine, and also requires energy to excrete excessive amounts via the kidney. The fat soluble vitamins, however, are more likely to cause serious toxicity, since they are more readily stored in the body. All vitamins are probably toxic in high quantities.

Megavitamin therapy has been well-received by the public, by physicians, and by those who wish to avoid certain drugs. Unfortunately the experimental data to support the efficacy of this kind of treatment is either non-existent, controversial, or open to varying interpretations. Megavitamin therapy seems to promise super health; and people falsely reason "If a little is good, a lot will be much better." The experiences of life, the mounting evidence from the investigation of degenerative disease, and extensive studies of food habits of large population groups who take no supplements, lead us to different conclusions. It is well-known that eating too little is wrong, eating an optimum amount is correct, and that eating more is damaging to the body. The principles of elementary pharmacology teach us that in any kind of theraputic regimen, increasing the dosage to maximum effectiveness is the objective. With further increases, serious toxic effects are usually produced. At higher than nutritional levels, vitamins have a pharmacodynamic effect. Any nutrient administered in a dosage exceeding 100% of the RDA should be considered a drug, not a nutrient. Several vitamins, including vitamins C and B-12, in high quantities may promote cancer.[123]

Uses of Vitamins

1. Vitamins promote the rate and ease with which essential chemical reactions proceed in the body, in much the same way that catalysts promote reactions in chemistry. True catalysts are not themselves used up in the reaction, whereas often the vitamins are used up, attached, or destroyed in the process of promoting the biologic reaction.

2. They regulate metabolism. Many of the vitamins are so essential to the regulation of metabolism that a particular process cannot occur in the body in the absence of the vitamin.

3. They assist in converting fat and carbohydrates into energy. In order for fats and carbohydrates to be quickly converted into energy, vitamins

are required. Carbohydrates follow the equation given below in turning the raw product into energy:

$$\text{Carbohydrate} + H_2O + O_2 + \text{B-vitamins} \xrightarrow[\text{Enzymes}]{\text{Certain}} \text{Energy} + CO_2 + H_2O$$

4. They assist in forming bones and tissue. There are many vitamins that are essential to the production of tissues, such as vitamin D in the formation of bones. It appears that all cells of the body, notably blood cells and gastrointestinal lining cells, require B-12.

5. They prevent deficiency diseases. One of the brightest chapters in medical history is that of the discovery of how to prevent pellagra, scurvy, rickets, night blindness, hemorrhagic diseases of the newborn, and beriberi. It seems incredible that less than a century ago, these diseases were widespread scourges of unknown cause.

Cooking Instructions for Vitamins

In order to minimize the losses of vitamins from fruits and vegetables during the cooking process, there are certain rules that should be carefully followed:

Little water. In cooking fruits and vegetables, vitamins can be leached from every cut surface and often through the skins of various fruits and vegetables. In order to minimize the losses of vitamins, little water should be used, and all that is left in the pot should be preserved and used in preparation of other food so that no essential nutrients will be lost.

Little time. The shortest possible exposure to heat should be used.

Little heat. Use the lowest level of heat that can accomplish the needed conversions in the proteins, carbohydrates, and structures of the various foods. Usually 212 degrees F. (100 degrees C.) is used, being most efficient and prompt in making these conversions. Cooking protein and carbohydrate foods increases their palatability, digestion, and absorption. However, heat damages certain vitamins to the point that they may no longer be useful to body systems.

Little air. The less exposure of cut surfaces to air, the better. Wilted, oxidized, and discolored foods are an indication that air and light may have damaged the food. Discoloration of bananas, apples, and potatoes on peeling produces very little nutrient loss and no known toxic substances.

Little chopping. Each cut surface is capable of large losses of the water soluble vitamins.

Avoid alkaline conditions. In an attempt to preserve the color of fruits or vegetables, alkaline substances such as baking soda are sometimes added during the cooking procedure. Such treatment causes a loss of nutrients.

Causes of Decreased Vitamin Absorption from the Gastrointestinal Tract

Mineral oil. The fat soluble vitamins can be dissolved in mineral oil, which is not broken down by the digestive enzymes. Bound to indigestible mineral oil, the fat soluble vitamins can pass out of the gastrointestinal tract in the fecal stream.

Antibiotics. Because antibiotics destroy the bacterial flora of the gastrointestinal tract, vitamins K, B-1, folacin, and B-12 can be reduced in quantity due to the loss of synthesis by microorganisms.

Drugs. Many drugs are capable of interfering with the absorption of various nutrients from the gastrointestinal tract. All drugs are irritating to the gastrointestinal tract. Through an irritation, the gastrointestinal tract may be made unhealthy, and thereby unable to absorb vitamins.

Certain Diseases. When the digestive tract is diseased the vitamins cannot be absorbed as well. Vitamin deficiency sometimes results. Sprue, celiac disease, ulcerative colitis, Crohn's disease, some parasitic infections (notably giardiasis), peptic ulcer, and other diseases are of this type.

An interesting problem may occur with anatomical conditions that promote stasis in the small bowel. The "blind loop syndrome" is increasingly seen due to the many surgical procedures done for peptic ulcer. In these procedures that create an intestinal pouch or blind loop, overgrowth of bacteria may occur. The bacteria then compete for vitamin B-12 and folacin, producing a deficiency state.

Stress. Because of altered motility of the gastrointestinal tract, a reduced production of digestive enzymes, or other factors, stress can cause a reduction in absorption from the gastrointestinal tract. Stress also causes an increase in the bowel metabolic rate which may cause an increase in the need for vitamins.

Multiple Combinations of Foods. Because of physical or chemical interactions, many foods compete with one another for absorption sites, or are absorbed or attached in such a way as to be unavailable for utilization or absorption.

Poor Chewing. The chemicals of digestion do not have ready access to all parts if the food is delivered to the stomach in large chunks. Food should be chewed to a cream in the mouth before it is swallowed.

"If your time to eat is limited, do not bolt your food, but eat less, and masticate slowly. The benefit derived from food does not depend so much on the quantity eaten as on its thorough digestion; nor the gratification of taste so much on the amount of food swallowed as on the length of time it remains in the mouth. Those who are excited, anxious, or in a hurry, would do well not to eat until they have found rest or relief; for the vital powers, already severely taxed, cannot supply the necessary digestive fluids."[124]

How the Body Uses Vitamins

Vitamin A is needed for maintaining normal mucous membranes, proper night vision, normal growth, and tissue repair. Deficiency can eventually lead to eye damage and blindness, loss of balance, decreased taste and smell thresholds, and thick scaling of the skin. Adequate vitamin A tends to inhibit cancer in animals. Vitamin A increases the defense mechanism against infections. A liberal intake over a long period has been found to increase longevity of animals and the vitality of the adults and offspring. Increased protein intake increases the need for vitamin A. Large doses of vitamins C and E are undesirable as they may reduce the availability of vitamin A in the body.

Vitamin A is highly toxic at doses not much higher than the recommended daily allowance as manifested by skin lesions, generalized itching, hair loss, blurred vision, and headache.

Vitamins A and C Content of Foods

Recommended Amounts per Day(National Research Council, 1979 Revision)

	Adult Men	Adult Women
Vitamin A (I.U.)	3000	2400
Vitamin C (I.U.)	50-60	60

Food	Size Portion	Vitamin A (I. U.)	Vitamin C (Mg)
Greens	3½ oz.	7,000	50
Cantaloupe	½ av. melon	6,200	60
Sweet potato	½ cup	8,800	21
Carrot	½ cup	11,000	8
Tomato	1 medium	1,640	8
Cabbage	1 c. shredded	80	50
Orange	1 medium	290	77
Grapefruit	½ medium	160	76
Strawberries	⅔ cup	60	59
Green peas	½ cup	640	20
Potato	1 medium	20	20

The B-vitamins, especially vitamin B-1, pantothenic acid, niacin, and B-12 are specifically nerve cell nutrients, just as iodine is a specific thyroid nutrient and vitamin A is a nutrient for the retina. Nerve cells develop severe abnormalities in microscopic appearance and in function when B-vitamins are deficient or lacking.

Vitamin B-1 (Thiamine)

This is the good disposition vitamin. The integrity of the central nervous system and the proper functioning of the gastrointestinal tract are associated with proper amounts of thiamine, along with all other B-vitamins. Thiamine serves an important function in maintaining normal appetite and digestion and is essential in carbohydrate metabolism and in the synthesis of acetylcholine (the nerve hormone that makes muscles move). A high level of mental function is not possible with a thiamine deficiency. Learning, praying, meditating, cheerfulness, being organized, and other heavy functions of the mind are reduced. Almost all natural foods contain thiamine. It is present in generous amounts in foods such as legumes, food yeast, whole grains, nuts, seeds, and grains. A thiamine deficiency leads to a disabling disease, beriberi, with stiffness, weakness, heart muscle injury, nerve deterioration, and absent tendon reflexes. It is characterized by tissue swelling, abnormally slow heart rate, congestive heart failure, loss of appetite, nausea, and inflamed or irritated nerves.

Thiamine-specific hunger has been demonstrated by thiamine deficient rats. In one experiment, the vitamin, when mixed with water and placed in cages, was quickly discovered by its odor, even when placed with as many as twelve other containers filled with different foods or solutions. The animals would hold onto bottles with both paws or even with the teeth, when researchers attempted to remove the bottle containing thiamine.

Chlorinated water destroys thiamine. Rice cooked in tap water had 36% less thiamine than rice cooked in distilled water.[125] Thiamine is lost in cooking at too high temperatures, cooking in an alkaline medium, and maintaining cooking temperatures for excessively long periods. Persons who rely on restaurants for their major food intake may be missing vitamins which are destroyed by prolonged exposure to heat, light, and air.

Vitamin B-2 (Riboflavin)

Riboflavin is present in leafy vegetables, whole

grain breads, and legumes. A deficiency of riboflavin causes lesions of the mouth; a smooth, painful tongue; hair loss; scaliness of the skin, with a flaking dermatitis between the nose and lip; and other skin lesions. Deficiency is rare except in gastrointestinal surgery or when the diet is extremely high in refined and concentrated foods, especially the so-called "empty calorie junk foods."

Pellagra

Pellagra is a disease due to deficiency of niacin, characterized by the "three D's": dermatitis, diarrhea, and dementia. It was a great and perplexing epidemic about 75 years ago before it was recognized that the cause is a vitamin deficiency. When diet was shown to be at the root of the disease, it was then called a disease of "three M's"—meat, meal, and molasses (where meat refers to pork and meal refers to corn meal). Since the amino acid tryptophan can be used to make niacin in the body, any food containing significant amounts of tryptophan will prevent pellagra. Corn is low in tryptophan and niacin. When corn forms a major part of the diet, as in Southeastern states during the winters of 90 years ago, pellagra can be expected to be fairly prevalent. The disease occurred in the spring and early summer after several winter months of the monotonous diet of corn grits and meal, cane syrup, and pork products. The meat in the diet was not conducive to good production of niacin by bacterial flora in the gastrointestinal tract, and the use of much syrup required increased niacin to convert the sugars in the diet into energy. This combination resulted in a high incidence of pellagra. Early symptoms of the disease are loss of appetite, weakness, and indigestion. A deficiency of any of the B-vitamins will give some kind of gastrointestinal symptoms.

The story is told of Dr. George Washington Carver, a professor from Tuskegee Institute, that he "saved the South" from pellagra. It is true that he put forth herculean efforts in that direction, even though he did not know the relationship between pellagra and niacin. He knew that people were healthier if they ate greens, and that collards grew luxuriantly in the South. Wherever he worked as a door to door health educator there was little or no pellagra. Dr. Carver would hitch up his buggy, place in it several large jars of collard seed from his own garden, and drive through the rural districts around Tuskegee Institute. He stopped all passersby, turned in at every home and in his quiet manner gave them a sample of the seed and brief instructions on cultivation and harvesting of collards. To this day in eastern Alabama the gardens behind the houses will be seen to contain tall, well-cropped collard stalks, a silent monument to the medical missionary work of a great American.

Niacin can be synthesized by certain bacteria in the intestine. Certain diets are more favorable for this synthesis than others, with a vegetarian diet being far more favorable than a meat-based diet. The tissues can synthesize niacin from tryptophan in a ratio of 60 mg. of tryptophan to 1 mg. of niacin. Legumes and nuts are good sources of tryptophan. All the niacin required to prevent pellegra can be made within the body if the diet is high in tryptophan. Foods from the vegetable kingdom contain more tryptophan than animal products.

In a test study, a direct correlation was observed between daily intake of tryptophan and the psychological state, with a better psychological state observed in those getting 1000 mg. of tryptophan per day or more.[126]

Vitamin	Function	Sources	Toxicity
A	Night vision, epithelial integrity, bone and tooth formation, mucus secretion, reproduction and lactation, prevention of xerophthalmia (inflammation and blindness).	Yellow and green vegetables and fruits. The deeper the color the more vitamin A.	Stunting of growth, bone fragility, loss of appetite, skin eruption, irritability and double vision, headaches, lethargy, ringing in the ears, muscle and joint pains, dry skin, sparse hair, anemia, low white blood cell count, and splenomegaly.
D	Formation of bones and teeth, maintenance of blood calcium, prevention of rickets (knockknees, soft bones, bowlegs, pigeon breast, bossing and beading of bones).	Sunshine, animal fats	Excessive calcium of bones, metastatic calcification, headaches, nausea, vomiting, diarrhea, and reduced growth.
E	Antioxidant, prevents peroxidation, retards aging, prevents one of the hemolytic anemias of the newborn.	Widely distributed	Depression of bone calcification and overall growth in chicks. Increase in time required for blood clotting.

E	Blood coagulation	Tomatoes, grains, cabbage, widely distributed	Hemolytic anemia
B complex	Need is determined by carbohydrate intake. Deficiency is a disease of food refining, bringing about certain deficiencies. Central nervous system stability, skin and epithelial integrity.	Greens, beans, whole grains, fruits, and vegetables.	Excesses of one may cause imbalances producing relative deficiencies of others, or of the one administered if it is suddenly decreased. Excessive doses of niacin can cause acanthosis nigricans, a precancerou condition. Excessive doses of B complex can destroy vitamin B-12. Large doses of nicotinic acid produce liver damage, as does B-6.
B-12	Blood formation, central nervous system integrity, gastrointestinal function. Hydrochloric acid is necessary to split from peptide bonds.	Greens, especially turnips, yeast, olives, soybeans, wheat, mouth and nasopharyngeal organisms, rain water, kelp, unsprayed fruit.	Cancer in animals from large doses, interference with utilization of other vitamins. Both B-12 and folic acid tend to aggravate seizures in some patients.* Folacin and intrinsic factor necessary for abundant absorption.
C	Intracellular cement, maintains collagen, prevents aging.	Raw fruits and vegetables, potatoes, cabbage, tomatoes. Not present in the skins of white or sweet potatoes as much as in the pulp.	Gastrointestinal irritation, interference in other vitamin balance, perhaps kidney oxalate stones. Overdose may cause altered copper metabolism, decreasing the amount that can be absorbed from food.

*Reynolds, E. H./ Modern Trends in Neurology. Fifth Edition. London: Butterworths, p. 276.

Vitamin B-6 (Pyridoxine)

Pyridoxine, or vitamin B-6, is active in the production of blood, in central nervous system metabolism, and in amino acid metabolism. Deficiencies may cause hemolytic anemias and convulsions. Oral contraceptives cause vitamin B-6 deficiency in about 25% of the users. Whole grain cereals, legumes, bananas, oatmeal, and potatoes are very good sources of B-6, and deficiencies other than in users of oral contraceptives are very rare.

Pantothenic Acid and Biotin

As its name implies, pantothenic acid is of such widespread occurrence in foods that deficiency states in humans are probably extremely rare. Dr. Roger Williams fed a group of dogs a diet lacking in pantothenic acid. They ate the diet for weeks and appeared healthy until a day or so before they suddenly died. The cells and tissues had become deficient, but the animals had continued to live until the heart muscle was starved to such an extent that it ceased to function.

Biotin, one of the B-complex group, is found in a wide variety of foods, especially yeast, soybeans, rice bran, and many other grains, fruits, and vegetables. Its deficiency is almost unknown in humans, except for rare reports of "egg-white injury," occurring in unusual individuals who subsist mostly on raw egg whites. The injury is due to avidin, a substance found in egg albumin, which binds biotin tightly and inactivates it. Avidin is destroyed by heat.

Vitamin C

Scurvy is a disease characterized by irritability, swollen and bleeding gums, dermatitis, weakness, prostration, and death. Vitamin C helps to maintain blood vessel integrity, assists in the absorption of iron and in the formation of hemoglobin, assists in resistance to infection and in wound healing, and is concerned with the manufacture of steroid hormones. Vitamin C is necessary to make collagen fibers, the framework for many tissues of the body. It has been shown that as little as ten milligrams of vitamin C daily can prevent the symptoms of scurvy. That would figure out to be about 1/6 of an orange daily. One small tangerine will have as much as 60 mg of vitamin C; one cooked potato as much as 30-50 mg. Vitamin C in usual dietary quantities increases the rate of degradation of cholesterol to bile acids and may therefore be a factor in prevention of atherosclerosis. Vitamin C protects against otherwise lethal effects of cadmium.

As with all nutrients there is an optimal level of intake; there is also that which is too little and that which is too much. In one study, high doses of vitamin C caused an increase in blood sugar in rats that persisted for three weeks. Excessive quantities of vitamin C can reduce the pH of the urine to as low as four, and cause the precipitation of large quantities of urates, increasing the risk of kidney stones. It appears that excessive doses of vitamin C interfere with purine metabolism, increasing the risk of gout. There is some evidence that high doses of vitamin C reduce fertility in some women. Vitamin C increases intestinal peristalsis and may produce diarrhea. This laxative action may be the source of any protective mechanism vitamin C may have against the common cold. Nausea and abdominal cramps may be a toxic sign.

Vitamin D

This vitamin is synthesized in the skin upon exposure to sunlight. The vitamin is intimately related to calcium metabolism, involving both absorption of calcium from the intestine and its use in the body. A deficiency of vitamin D leads to rickets, a disease in which the bones do not form properly, resulting in such conditions as knock-knees, bow legs, and pigeon breast. Since phytates in unleavened breads have been questioned as being the cause of some cases of rickets, as they are believed to interfere with calcium, iron, and possibly zinc absorption, a study was done to test whether rickets is more common in those who use large quantities of unleavened bread. It was determined that rickets developing in dark-skinned Asians living in the United Kingdom is due to the lack of sunlight or vitamin D in the diet, as unleavened breads did not seem to make any difference in the progress of the disease or its resolution. It is concluded that unleavened chapattis, with their high phytate content, have no effect on the development of rickets.[127]

Persons who live in smog laden air must put forth special effort to avoid any threat of vitamin D deficiency, particularly in dark-skinned children living in geographic areas subject to long periods of cloudy skies day after day. Children are more susceptible to serious injury from vitamin D deficiency, as their bones can be permanently deformed if the deficiency occurs while the bones are being formed. Vitamin D is readily stored in the body, and children should obtain a long exposure to sunlight on every sunny day in winter, even fully clothed. In summer, children should store plenty of vitamin D if they live in areas which are cold, and cloudy in winter.

Vitamin E (Tocopherol)

Vitamin E is so prevalent in nearly every food man consumes that it is quite unlikely that a vitamin E deficiency could arise. The few deficiency states reported have involved infants fed certain prepared formulas that were deficient in vitamin E. Of course, breast feeding precludes deficiency from this source. Vitamin E is the most widely available of any of the vitamins in common foods. Green plants, grains, nuts, legumes, various seeds, fruits, and vegetables all contain vitamin E. It is completely fat-soluble, and boiling does not affect its potency. It is stored for long periods in adipose tissue and turns over very slowly in the body. Many months of deprivation would be required to deplete the body stores.

Vitamin E reacts with free radicals (harmful compounds that have unpaired electrons). A major source of fat-soluble free radicals is cooking oil (polyunsaturated fat) that has undergone oxidative deterioration, as after long storage or repeated deep fat frying. Vitamin E, functioning as an antioxidant, converts the free radical into a less reactive and less harmful form. This prevents the accumulation of free radicals which result from peroxidation processes in cells. It spares the polyunsaturated fats from oxidative deterioration and the other parts of the cell from free radical damage. Products of oxidative deterioration accumulate in the cells as pigments, such as lipofuscin. Vitamin E and other antioxidants protect against the storage of this aging pigment. Large losses of vitamin E occur in milling of grains and in freezing foods.

Depression of growth and bone calcification in chicks have been described as symptoms of vitamin E toxicity. Some recent studies have revealed a relationship between vitamin E and blood clotting time. Large doses of the vitamin increase the time required for blood to clot. This may have clinical significance for women taking oral contraceptives, who are at risk of developing thrombosis, and probably require more vitamin E from their normal food sources.[128,129,130]

Vitamin B-12

It has been believed that only animal products contain sufficient quantities of vitamin B-12 to meet human needs. This is not the case, and many pure vegetarians live a lifetime without evidence of B-12 deficiency. We believe that if it is searched for the cause of B-12 deficiency can always be found in some other quarter than the absence of animal products in the diet. Some of these matters will be briefly presented.

We should point out that B-12 deficiency is a very rare disorder, and the overwhelming majority of cases occur in non-vegetarians. Until the last few years, dietary deficiency of B-12 had never been considered as a cause of cellular deficiency. Mal-absorption, increased need, or increased elimination have been accepted as the most likely causes of a cellular deficiency of B-12. Known causes of B-12 malabsorption are a lack of intrinsic factor and hydrochloric acid in the stomach, the removal or disease of the second portion of the ileum, and competition for B-12 by microorganisms or intestinal parasites. Other causes are suspected, among them toxic substances. There is far more unknown than is known about B-12 and its meta-bolism in the body.

Vitamin B-12 was isolated in 1948. Merck and Company is the holder of various patents of pro-cedures for producing B-12 and owns the product claim. In 1951, 48 pounds of vitamin B-12 were pro-duced with a sales value of eleven million dollars. In 1952, 94 pounds were produced.

Non-Animal Sources of B-12

There are several vegetarian food sources of B-12. While these sources may not be constant, it ap-pears that they occur with sufficient frequency to supply the minute quantities of B-12 that are needed by those who are not abusing their health. These include wheat, soybeans, various common greens, olives, fruits, and many other foods that oc-casionally have B-12 either in or on the food.[131] Vita-min B-12 has been found in roots and stems of tomatoes, cabbage, celery, kale, broccoli, and leeks. It has been found in the leaves of kohlrabi.[132] Sea weed[133] and alfalfa[134] contain B-12. It is difficult to avoid B-12. One laboratory worker "found that it was necessary to acid-wash all pipettes, test tubes, and volumetric flasks and rinse them 15 times with tap water and 2 times with distilled water" in order to make her determinations for B-12 accurate. In her laboratory, the de-ionized water was found fre-quently to be a source of B-12.[135]

A further source of B-12 is bacterial growth in the mouth (around the teeth and gums), in the nasopharynx, around the tonsils and tonsillar crypts, in the folds at the base of the tongue, and in the upper bronchial tree. Up to 0.5 micrograms daily can be obtained from this source. It is likely that

this source alone will supply sufficient quantities of B-12 for the very small requirement that a pure vegetarian has, especially considering his low protein intake which further reduces the need for B-12.

It has also been shown that some bacteria which may colonize the small intestine of man can synthesize considerable amounts of biologically ac-tive forms of the vitamin.[136] The terminal ileum is principally involved in absorbing B-12. Since bac-teria can form B-12 above the terminal ileum, and since intrinsic factor which is needed for most rapid absorption is found in the ileum, there may be adequate absorption of vitamin B-12 produced from these bacteria in the ileum in many healthy people.

It is only a matter of time until all people will recognize that milk and eggs are unsafe to eat. It is not necessary for normal people to have them to obtain a supply of B-12, as it is quite possible to ob-tain all elements on nutrition from fruits, vegetables, and whole grains. Many population groups have al-ready demonstrated the feasibility of such a diet. This is not a new thing, but has been going on for centuries. Many of these population groups live in areas where population explosions are current, demonstrating that a simple diet does not reduce fertility or result in early death.

B-12 Supplements

Generally the routine use of vitamin B-12 supple-ments is not advised. In animal studies, there have been cases of increased cancer production in animals receiving high levels of B-12. It has been noted that the animals have an increased produc-tion of white blood cells such as occurs in chronic myelogenous leukemia. A case has been reported of acute myeloblastic leukemia resulting from B-12 overdosage in the treatment of pernicious anemia.[137] A group of French investigators reported a series of cases suggesting that B-12 may stimulate multipli-cation of cancer cells and aggravate the disease. Certainly, there is experimental evidence that B-12 encourages cell division in general and certain tumor cells in particular.[138]

Patients with rheumatoid arthritis present serum B-12 levels significantly higher than normal subjects.[139] It is also known to be higher in patients with ulcerative colitis, leukemia, and other serious illnesses. A high serum B-12 level should be a signal for a thorough medical evaluation.

The development of pernicious anemia and related metabolic states is not a simple or well understood subject. It is known that both absorption and conservation of B-12 are more important than its presence in the diet. In order to encourage best absorption and conservation of all nutrients, including B-12, gastrointestinal malfunction should be kept to a minimum. To accomplish this, one should pay close attention to the physiologic principles of digestion. These include using the proper combination of foods (avoiding milk-egg-sugar or fruit-vegetable combinations at the same meal); all major food eaten early in the day (morning food is more nourishing than the same food taken in the evening); keeping the varieties of food served at one meal to two or three dishes with bread; avoiding concentrated foods having high nutrient or caloric density; as well as carefulness in eating slowly and chewing well.

B-12 Requirements

Individuals taking conventional diets need only about 0.1 micrograms of B-12 per day,[140] even though conventional diets contain excesses of fat, animal protein, and refined foods, all of which increase the need for B-12.[141, 142, 143] In London, twelve vegans ranging in age from 18 to 71 were studied for physical defects referable to their "rigid" diets, which they had pursued for 4 to 30 years. It was discovered that five had B-12 levels in the normal range (140-900 pg/ml). The remaining seven had values so low as to suggest the diagnosis of pernicious anemia or subacute combined deterioration of the cord. Only three of the twelve admitted to any symptoms whatever, but it was felt by the investigators that it was possible that two of these may have had mild cases of combined degeneration of the cord. It is noteworthy that both of these were smokers.[144]

In pregnancy, the level of serum vitamin B-12 is lower in women who smoke than in non-smokers. This finding may be an effect of the cyanide content of tobacco smoke, which may be detoxified by a mechanism that depletes the stores of vitamin B-12 in the body.[145, 146, 147]

Vegans who have previously had an omnivorous diet will smile at the use of the word "rigid" in the above report. Most vegans declare their diets and menus to be more varied, more interesting, flavorful, and colorful since adopting a vegan menu. Yet, their food costs less in both preparation time and money spent. Gone forever are the days the cook pleads with the family to give her some suggestions

for a meal. When something is finally suggested other members state: "Oh, let's not have that again." Most vegans find the menu hard to control only because of the large number of delightful dishes one is tempted to put on the table (an unhealthful practice).

It is quite likely that vegan diets would require no more than 0.05 micrograms of B-12 daily. Breast-fed infants get only a tiny fraction of a microgram of B-12 per day, even if their mothers are on a high intake. Yet, they can build neurologic tissue, convert their hemoglobin from F to A type, and do many other complex functions believed to be dependent on B-12. Non-smoking vegans may not need any B-12 as such in their diets, as they apparently conserve B-12 avidly or develop the capacity to absorb adequate amounts of their bacterial production of B-12. An ounce of the roots of leeks, beets, and other vegetables will provide 0.1 to 0.3 micrograms of B-12, which is more than a day's supply. It has been suggested that in man, the normal requirement of B-12 is met by bacterial synthesis in the colon.[148, 149, 150] Many foods available to vegetarians contain from 1 to 50 micrograms of B-12 per 100 grams of food.[151]

The terminal ileum is apparently not the only source of absorption of B-12. Vitamin B-12 can be absorbed by inhalation.[152] While tests for absorption of B-12 from the human colon have not demonstrated its absorption,[153] this possibility cannot be excluded in the properly primed vegetarian after several years of a vegetarian diet.

Factors Affecting B-12 Deficiency

We do not require large quantities of B-12 unless certain conditions exist:

1. The body is habituated to large quantities of vitamin B-12.
2. Meat or other animal products and refined carbohydrates are used generously which may more than double B-12 needs.
3. The person uses drugs, chemicals, or beverages which destroy B-12 (nicotine, alcohol, caffeine, etc.)
4. The person takes multivitamin preparations containing B-12 (see discussion below).
5. A disease exists such as pernicious anemia, atherosclerosis, or diabetes which causes malnutrition.
6. Excessively high or low blood levels exist of other nutrients, most notably protein,[154] vitamin C, and calcium.

7. Oral contraceptives are used.

8. The person is very old or has a condition such as liver disease, tuberculosis, or other chronic infection; cancer, or previous surgery of the stomach or small bowel.

9. Intestinal parasites or malaria are present.

10. The thyroid function is low.

Rainwater has been found to be a source of vitamin B-12.[155] Spinach, amaranth, and alfalfa leaves have been shown to contain trace quantities of material having activity resembling that of vitamin B-12.[156,157]

Alkali-resistant thermostable factor (ARF) appears to have distinct capabilities of promoting blood formation. It is not known if ARF is a vitamin or if it is a natural factor found in the liver. It was first discovered during studies of B-12. It has been proven not to be a derivative of B-12. One microgram of the substance was effective in pernicious anemia, and a fifty-fold increase in dosage produced a response in folic acid deficiency anemia. It may be that ARF offers protection against neurological complications associated with pernicious anemia. Since ARF corrects anemia due to B-12 and folic acid deficiency, it may be that it has a place in the production metabolic pathways ordinarily controlled by B-12.[158]

High doses of vitamin C, as popularly used in home remedies for the common cold, destroy substantial amounts of vitamin B-12.[159] Vitamin C in quantities in excess of a half a gram will destroy 50-95% of B-12 content in food.[160] Megadoses of vitamin C may produce B-12 deficiency by destroying the cobalamins during transport through the gastrointestinal tract, and possibly also in the tissues.[161] Large doses of vitamin B-1 can also destroy vitamin B-12.

Multivitamin preparations contain breakdown products of B-12 that exert an anti-B-12 effect, and may cause the very deficiency the preparation is expected to prevent. Dr. Victor Herbert reported that all 10 of the multivitamin-mineral preparations they tested showed the anti-B-12 breakdown products. Tests for B-12 levels in the blood do not discriminate between the true vitamin B-12 and its breakdown products, therefore giving a false sense of security in cases who may be suffering from anemia due to a lack of the true B-12.[162]

Egg albumin and egg yolk decrease B-12 absorption.[163] A 20% soybean protein diet increased the fecal excretion of vitamin B-12.[164] There is a possibility that soybeans, particularly uncooked soybean products, may increase the excretion of B-

12. The use of oral contraceptives reduces the level of B-12 in the serum because of a change in B-12 binders of serum. Levels of thiamin, riboflavin, B-6, C, and folacin are also reduced.[165] A lactose intolerance may increase B-12 needs.[166]

Dietary Deficiency of Vitamin B-12

"Though strict vegetarians commonly have subnormal serum vitamin B-12 concentrations, dietary B-12 deficiency producing megaloblastic anemia is extremely rare."[167]

Almost all investigators reporting on the dietary habits of vegetarians and vegans mention mild changes, if any. Generally, they describe the followers of vegan diets as being unusually active and healthy, much above average. Some investigators report "mild megaloblastic anemia," in the area of 11 to 13 grams (!), with "early neurological complications." The use of the terms "anemia" and "megaloblastic" in reference to these individuals is highly questionable. It is a fact that nobody anywhere knows the ideal size of a red blood cell, and it can be successfully argued that the most efficient size of a red blood cell is that seen in vegans, and the most efficient hemoglobin level is 11 to 13. Investigation reveals this range to best promote wound healing,[168] childbirth without complications,[169] and a sense of well being into an advanced age. These statements are made in reference even to individuals who have been vegans for 30 to 50 years.[170, 171] Neurological deficits are rarely enumerated in the reports, and most of the reported individuals are elderly. Since mild neurological signs are almost universal with advancing age in all segments of the population, one suspects that elderly vegetarians may not have as many neurologic changes as the elderly on a mixed diet; certainly that is our experience. Sometimes very small population samples are used, inadequate to make a proper judgment. "Twenty-five selected patients cannot be assumed to be representative of about 1,000,000 immigrants from a sub-continent, let alone 'non-caucasian' races."[172]

When vegans in advanced old age are studied, they show no more signs of B-12 deficiency than others. Most vegans who have been on the diet for 16 to 50 years are in excellent health, with no symptoms detectable.[173] Red blood cell indices, mean corpuscular hemoglobin and mean corpuscular volume are both higher, but within normal range for vegans as compared to controls, regardless of whether or not they take B-12 supplements.[174]

Malabsorption of B-12

If there is not enough B-12 absorbed into the blood, the body begins to make large but ineffective red blood cells. There are problems with digestion and sometimes signs of nerve degeneration. The skin may develop dark, pigmented patches. These symptoms[175] are called pernicious anemia. The typical patient is tall, blue-eyed, has large ears, and premature graying of the hair. The patient is more likely to be male and of Northern European background. Negros rarely have pernicious anemia. These patients often have antibodies against their gastric lining cells. It may be that the atrophic changes in the stomach lining depend on an auto-immune reaction.[176] Pernicious anemia has no relationship to dietary intake of B-12.

Chewing properly, leaving plenty of time between meals, and not eating large varieties of food at any one meal are important for encouraging absorption of B-12, especially if the pancreas is functioning poorly. The influence of saliva on B-12 is a beneficial one, binding it in such a way that it apparently is more usable by the body's tissues.[177, 178] Possession of this knowledge enables us to promote more vigorously the practice of long and thorough chewing of one's food. In certain studies, absorption of B-12 was decreased by charcoal, but not by bile or saliva.[179]

CHAPTER NINE

Minerals

Mineral Content of the Body

Organic chemicals are those produced by a living organism. Inorganic chemicals are those that occur naturally; they are not made secondarily by a living organism. There are seventeen minerals, inorganic chemicals, proven essential for man, but more than twenty have been found in human ash:

Al	Aluminum	**Mg**	Magnesium
Sb	Antimony	**Mn**	Manganese
As	Arsenic	**Mo**	Molybdenum
Ba	Barium	**Ni**	Nickel
Bi	Bismuth	**P**	Phosphorus
Br	Bromine	**K**	Potassium
Ca	Calcium	**Se**	Selenium
Cl	Chlorine	**Si**	Silicon
Cr	Chromium	**Ag**	Silver
Co	Cobalt	**Na**	Sodium
Cu	Copper	**Sr**	Strontium
F	Fluorine	**S**	Sulfur
Ga	Gallium	**Sn**	Tin
I	Iodine	**V**	Vanadium
Fe	Iron	**Zn**	Zinc

The percentage of body weight occupied by various chemicals is as follows:

Oxygen	65%	Minerals	4%
Carbon	18%		
Hydrogen	10%		
Nitrogen	3%		
Total gases in compounds	96%	Total Solids	4%
(144 pounds in a 150 pound man)		(6 pounds in a 150 pound man)	

Uses in the Body

No element can function in any way, be deficient or in surplus without affecting all other elements in the body. Minerals can be imbalanced by the way we eat or by failure to get sufficient exercise.

Minerals serve very important functions in the metabolic economy. They maintain an acid-base balance in the body by shifting easily into plasma or out of plasma into bone or muscle. Minerals slide around readily to provide the narrow tolerance we have for a change in acids or bases in blood or tissues. Minerals can be hitched to acids or bases and quickly poured out in the urine. This important function of minerals is one on which life is based.

Minerals help to maintain osmotic pressure. Probably everyone has had the experience of eating too much salt, and retaining fluid in fingers, face, or feet. Fluids shift readily to accompany minerals. We can say that where there is a grain of salt, there must be a drop of water.

Minerals facilitate transport across cell membranes. There are some mechanisms, such as the sodium pump, that are used mainly for minerals, but can be shared by other nutrients to get across cell membranes. Minerals provide a medium for nerve transmission and muscle contraction. Our Designer used an enormously complicated system of shifting sodium, potassium, chloride, calcium, and various hormones and enzymes to make it possible for us to use flesh to carry electrical currents and do mechanical labor.

Minerals assist in blood clotting. Calcium is essential for blood clotting as also are other minerals. One of the most important minerals is calcium; yet, in excess it is injurious to tissues, just as is the essential mineral, sodium.

Minerals make up a significant portion of the bony skeleton and teeth. Hard compounds are made by the formation of calcium salts which give structure to the rigid parts of the body.

Requirements

When calories, proteins, and vitamins are provided in sufficient quantity by a varied diet from the basic three food groups, the mineral requirements are usually met automatically. It is not helpful to any of the body systems to have a mineral surplus on hand. In fact, body functions are hampered or even destroyed by an excess.

Pica

Pica is an unnatural craving seen commonly in women and young children. Persons who exhibit this condition eat such materials as laundry starch, clay, ashes, dirt, ice, or similar materials. It is probably due in part to a natural craving for trace minerals, especially iron. Pagophagia, ice eating, is characteristic of iron deficiency anemia. Pica may be seen during pregnancy or lactation. The presence of the materials eaten may prevent absorption of vital nutrients such as iron and produce serious deficiencies.

Specific Minerals

Calcium. In addition to its function in the blood clotting mechanism, calcium is used in enzymatic activity and stabilization of enzyme systems, for permeability of cell membranes, for nerve transmission and muscle responsiveness, and to provide the mineral matrix for bones and teeth.

If there is too wide a variety of elements in any part of the intestine, calcium may be precipitated and become unusable. Calcium must be in a water soluble form in order to be utilized. Some salts that precipitate out of the gastrointestinal tract are then insoluble in water, and therefore, unusable. This principle was recognized by Ellen G. White about 100 years ago. She spoke of the "war" inside the body from too many varieties of food. "In all the restaurants in our cities, there is danger that the combinations of many foods in the dishes served shall be carried too far. The stomach suffers when so many kinds of food are placed in it at one meal....

If the patronage of our restaurants lessens because we refuse to depart from right principles, then let it lessen. We must keep the way of the Lord through evil report as well as good report."[180]

A high protein-diet causes man's body to lose calcium. This loss does not occur on a moderate or low-protein diet. Experimental studies on college men at Wisconsin Agricultural Experiment Station showed that a high protein diet (142 gram daily) caused the loss of excessive quantities of calcium in the urine. Even with extra calcium added to the diet to make calcium intake 1400 mg per day, the losses continued. A normal protein intake (47 gm), however, showed no adverse effect on calcium imbalance in the body. Both groups were eating the same food except for the supplemental protein in the diet of the one group.

Only 20-30% of calcium is ordinarily absorbed from food. Calcium overload is toxic to the body. Therefore, a barrier mechanism for preventing the over-absorption from food has been designed by an all wise Creator. Vitamin D helps metabolize calcium that the body cannot use. It helps the intestine absorb calcium five to fifty times better. If 100% of calcium were taken up from the food, most people would develop toxicity. During pregnancy, when the need is greater, 40% of the calcium present in food may be asorbed. During infancy and early childhood, 65% or more may be absorbed.

Calcium is the most abundant mineral in the body. Its absorption is controlled by the intestine partly by need. Calcium absorption is increased by the activity of the gastric juice. The formation of lactose-calcium complexes increases the absorption of calcium, a feature making it possible for infants to absorb a greater amount during their greater need. Exercise also increases the absorption of calcium.[181, 182] The reversal of the factors which increase absorption of calcium will, of course, depress its absorption as will a high intake of oxalic acid. Calcium may be precipitated into insoluble forms by certain other dietary constituents. Oxalic acid in the diet may form calcium oxalate, an insoluble salt. Certain greens contain significant quantities of oxalic acid. These are spinach, swiss chard, beet tops, wild poke and rhubarb. Most of these greens contain a large amount of calcium, and the end result is that not much calcium is moved either way, into or out of the body. The oxalic acid ties up its own calcium in the greens but does not remove stored calcium from the body. These greens cannot, therefore, be depended on to yield much calcium to the diet, even though the analysis reports a high content of calcium in them. The simple addition of rice to the diet apparently corrects part of the problem caused by oxalate according to feeding experiments, producing proper utilization of calcium from greens containing oxalate. [183, 187]

Phytic acid, found in the outer husks of grains, especially oats, will depress absorption of calcium.[184,185,186] However, the enzyme phytase is produced by the body in response to frequent exposure to phytic acid, greatly nullifying its binding effect. Less calcium is absorbed when there is rapid digestion (decreased transit time), stress, or an increase in the phosphorus level. Calcium enhances the absorption of vitamin D, fats and proteins.

Calcium in Common Foods

Food Source	Quantity	Calories	Protein gm	Carbohydrate gm	Fat gm	Sodium mg	Calcium mg
Human breast milk	1 cup	184	2.4	22.4	9.6	40	80
Cow's milk							
Whole, fresh	1 cup	159	8.5	12.0	8.6	122	288
Nonfat, skim	1 cup	88	8.8	12.6	.2	128	298
Nonfat, skim, fortified	1 cup	105	9.8	13.6	1.2	142	359
Soy milk							
Soyagen, all purpose	1 cup	146	7.3	11.0	8.5	303	72
Soyamel, all purpose	1 cup	140	5.0	16.0	6.0	363	150
Broccoli, cooked	1 cup	32	4.1	60	4	13	117
Collards, cooked	1 cup	58	5.4	9.8	1.2	50	304
Lambsquarters, cooked	1 cup	64	6.4	10.0	1.4		516
Mustard greens, cooked	1 cup	46	4.4	8.0	.8	36	278
Sesame seed, whole	2 T	125	4.1	4.8	10.9	13	258
Sunflower seed kernels	2 T	124	5.3	4.4	10.5	6.7	27
Soybeans, cooked	1 cup	260	22.0	21.6	11.4	4	146
Kale, cooked	1 cup	48	4.3	7.5	1.0	94	224
Oatmeal cereal, cooked	1 cup	123	5.6	23.3	0.8	169	191
Cream of wheat, cooked	1 cup	130	4.4	26.9	0.4	96	185

For adults with a protein intake as low as the current RDA (56 gm for men, 46 gm for women), many nutritionists believe 350 mg of calcium daily would be adequate, rather than the allowance of 800 mg per day recommended in 1968. This recommended level of calcium is well above that of Canada, the United Kingdom, and FAO/WHO.[188]

It may be taken as a biologic law that the body utilizes material more efficiently when in need. Macy showed that three boys fed a standard diet could retain an average of 374 mg of calcium per day. A similar group of boys who had received a high calcium diet for approximately two months prior to the experimental period, although on the same diet as the others, retained only 103 mg of calcium per day.[189]

The lesson here is that those on a rich dietary will tend to excrete more calcium because it is not needed, whereas, those on a more "prudent" diet, who take in less calcium, will tend to utilize it more fully and excrete less. In fact, because calcium is toxic in overdosage, and conversely a deficiency results in poor bodily performance, the built-in barriers and enhancers can be seen to be essential to proper order in a system based on random food selection. It is growing more apparent that the emphasis we have placed on calcium in the past is ill-advised, since the body is quite capable of regulating its uptake from a reasonable diet based on its need. If a simple, varied, and wholesome diet is taken, not rich or refined, the calcium needs will be amply supplied. Men have the ability to adapt to calcium intakes as low as 200-400 mg daily.[190]

The fact that human milk contains only 80 mg of calcium per cup, as compared to 288 mg per cup for dairy milk, should give us confidence that humans do not require the large quantities of calcium provided by dairy milk. During the most rapid growth period of a child, the only food supply should be nothing but human milk. This fact provides an indication that the amount of calcium needed during childhood and youth is far below that usually recommended, based on dairy milk values. As a general rule, vegetarian children do not have as many broken bones or carious teeth as children given a mixed dietary with generous quantities of dairy milk.

Excess calcium in the diet endangers many tissues from "metastatic" calcium deposition in such organs and tissues as kidneys, gallbladder, arteries, heart valves, joints, muscles, and skin. The dietary emphasis is better placed on variety, wholesomeness, simplicity, and naturalness; not on enrichment or concentration.

Sodium. There is a steady state between the intake of sodium and its excretion in sweat, urine, and feces. No dietary allowances have been set, because the normal diet generally provides an excess of sodium, and its use needs to be curbed. Canners of baby food add salt greatly increasing the sodium intake of small children. Babies will accept their food perfectly well without salt if they have not been trained to expect it. In contrast to breast milk, dairy milk contains high levels of sodium.

There is an exceptional loss of sodium through sweating, vomiting, and excretion of large volumes of urine. Deficiency symptoms such as nausea, vertigo, muscular weakness, and respiratory failure are non-specific. When too much sodium accumulates in the blood or tissues, there is retention of water and possibly an increase in blood pressure. The common foods that are highest in sodium are milk and dairy products; meat, especially the processed types; most baked goods (due to added salt, baking powder, and baking soda); and canned vegetables (due to added salt). Detergents, ion-exchange filters, toothpaste, a large number of drugs, and many other sodium sources add some sodium bit by bit to the total intake of this mineral. As many of these sources should be avoided as possible in a salt free diet.

Iron. Hemoglobin, the blood protein that carries oxygen, is the major iron-containing compound in humans. Foods that are high in iron include green leafy vegetables, legumes, prunes, dried apricots, raisins, nuts, and whole grains. Peaches, dried apricots, and prunes are most active in raising the hemoglobin. Raisins, grapes, and apples are next. Berries, except for blackberries and blueberries, are not helpful. The enrichment of flour and bread with vitamins and iron has been practiced since around 1940. While there is much controversy about what constitutes "simple iron deficiency anemia," there continues to be considerable concern about hemoglobins that are believed to be too low. This has been the initiating factor in the decision to enrich wheat flour, farina, bread, buns, and rolls with iron. There are many enriched and unenriched wheat-based products available in today's market place. Enriched products are clearly labled as such. About 85-90% of all white bread consumed in the United States is enriched; 10-15% is unenriched. Whole wheat bread, rye bread, and raisin bread are unenriched.

A serious question must be faced when ·any decision to enrich food is made: Is there a likelihood of toxicity to any segment of our population resulting from the enrichment program? The possibility of iron overload has been studied at some length and is a definite risk, especially for men who tend to eat more bread, retain more iron, and suffer more consistently from polycythemia or hemochromatosis than do women.[191] Both of these diseases are life-threatening. In contrast, the role in women of a "low" hemoglobin of 10 grams or even below in producing symptoms of lack of vitality or of increasing susceptibility to infection is far from proven. It is probable that 10.5 to 12.5 grams of hemoglobin are ideal for women living below 5,000 feet elevation.

So called "iron deficient" Somali nomads were divided into two groups, 67 given a placebo and 71 given iron. There were only seven episodes of infection in the placebo group as compared to 36 in the iron treated group. The 36 episodes included tuberculosis, brucellosis, and activation of pre-

existing malaria. The host defense was greater against infections when the hemoglobins were in the range we have customarily called anemia. The investigators used as criteria for iron deficiency a hemoglobin of less than 11 gm/dl, a serum iron concentration less than 25 ug/100ml, a transferrin saturation of less than 15%, and a peripheral blood smear showing small, pale cells (microcytic hypochromasia).[192]

Heavy blood puts an extra burden on the heart and blood vessels. As the blood gets thicker, the blood pressure goes up.[193]

It has been shown that an elevated hemoglobin can cause failure in surgery in a diabetic foot. Eighteen amputations done on diabetic patients with preoperative hemoglobin values less than 12 were successful, while 30 amputations in those whose hemoglobin was greater than 13 failed.[194] The results are just opposite to what surgeons have customarily understood, a patient often being transfused if the hemoglobin measured less than 12 gm.

"There is insufficient knowledge of the effects of mild iron deficiency to warrant the statement that iron deficiency anemia is a major nutritional problem in the United States."[195] Enriching bread with iron may have the ill effect of making certain diseases, such as chronic bleeding from cancer of the colon or from peptic ulcer, more difficult to diagnose. Many of those opposed to iron enrichment believe that it would be prudent to wait until adequate data is available so that a convincing risk-benefit ratio can be determined.

Since excess iron can injure the body, just as with calcium, there is a mechanism designed by an All-wise Creator, for preventing over-absorption of this mineral. The intestine itself possesses the mechanism to prevent too much iron absorption. Less than 10% of dietary iron is usually absorbed by an adult. A further mechanism preventing the excessive absorption of iron is that it forms insoluble compounds with other dietary substances, as does calcium. Phytates from whole grains, calcium, phosphates, copper, zinc, cadmium, and antacids are all known to tie up iron. If tissues become depleted, however, a person can absorb as much as 30% or more of dietary iron. If the hemoglobin goes down too far, the disorder is termed anemia. When the body stores of iron become depleted as from chronic gastrointestinal bleeding or excessive menstruation, it often takes years before these stores are replenished, even on a good diet.

Anemia is of three different types. The first is a nutritional deficiency, usually of iron, protein, copper, niacin, folacin, and very rarely B-6 and B-12. Chronic blood loss can cause iron deficiency anemia. Various malabsorption syndromes previously mentioned may interfere with absorption of iron, B-12, and folacin producing various deficiency-state anemias.

Excessive blood destruction is a second cause of anemia. Increased blood destruction comes from such disorders as hemolytic anemia, which can be due to exposure to toxic chemicals or may be related to certain diseases of the blood-forming organs. Viral infections can cause a drop of 1-2 grams of hemoglobin in only a day or two. The common cold or influenza can produce such reductions. Rarely, hereditary causes are at the root of excessive blood destruction.

A third cause of anemia is depression of the bone marrow. This condition is due to toxicity or hypersensitivity, as from the taking of certain drugs and other toxic substances or from chronic kidney disease.

The average person can correct certain types of anemia by simple remedies in the home. Of course, the usual program of good health carries a premium in anemia. Drink plenty of water: generally two glasses before breakfast, two mid-morning, two mid-afternoon, and one or two at night. Get adequate rest for body repair and rebuilding of blood cells. Fatigue causes poor blood. Eight hours of sleep each day is about right for most adults. Too much sleep is also improper. Avoid nervous tension. Remember that "Exercise neutralizes tension." Exercise also stimulates the bone marrow to produce blood cells, and is one of the most important treatments for anemia. Absorption of iron from the intestine is promoted by exercise. Low tissue levels of oxygen that occur during exercise lead to the production by the liver of erythropoitin which stimulates the bone marrow to produce red blood cells.

Sunshine stimulates blood-making. It promotes good health. Vitamin D assists in the making of blood, and can be obtained in adequate quantities from daily sun exposure of a six-inch square of skin. Good posture and deep breathing of pure air is a good way to build and to nourish all cells of the body. It is a natural protection against anemia.

Proper clothing of the extremities keeps the circulation equalized between the trunk and extremities. Proper blood building can be accomplished only by healthy bone marrow activity. Congestion of the trunk by blood which should be more equally distributed inhibits proper functioning of the bone marrow in the flat bones, where blood cells are manufactured. Habitual chilling of the extremities causes a tax on the body.

Chronic blood loss, as from excessive menstruation or a little daily loss from a bleeding point in the gastrointestinal tract, can keep the iron stores low. These conditions should be promptly corrected by proper measures.

Dietary factors that promote development of anemia start with a diet low in iron-containing foods. Women in particular are prone to take a diet low in iron. When coupled with menstrual losses, the stage is set for low iron stores. Excesses of calcium and phosphate salts inhibit the absorption of iron from the intestine. Milk is high in both these nutrients. Therefore, in anemia, it is well to avoid dairy products, as they contain very little iron, and tend to bind iron present in other foods.

The preparation of food in iron cookware "enriches" the food. As an example: It was found that a 100 gram serving of spaghetti sauce prepared in iron cookware contained 87.5 milligrams of iron compared to only three when cooked in a glass vessel.[196] Grandmother may have reared her strong, ruddy, and robust daughters on this kind of food enrichment program (less expensively, too).

Foods High in Iron*

Food	Weight Gm	Approximate Measure	Per Serving	Per 100 Gm
Almonds	15	12-15	0.7	4.4
Apricots, dried	30	5 halves	1.5	4.9
Bacon, cooked	25	4-5 slices	0.8	3.3
Beans, dried	30 (dry)	½ cup (cooked)	2.1	6.9
Lima, dried	30 (dry)	½ cup (cooked)	2.3	7.5
Beet greens, cooked	75	½ cup	2.4	3.2
Brazil nuts	15	2 medium	0.5	3.4
Breaded, whole wheat	25	1 slice	0.6	2.2
Cashews	15	6-8	0.8	5.0
Chard	75	½ cup	1.9	2.5
Coconut, fresh	15	½ ounce	0.3	2.0
Dried	15	2 tablespoons	0.5	3.6
Cornmeal, degermed, enriched	15 (dry)	½ cup (cooked)	0.4	2.9
Cress, garden	10	5-8 sprigs	0.3	2.9
Currants, dried	30	2 tablespoons	0.8	2.7
Dandelion greens	75	½ cup	2.3	3.1
Dates	30	3-4	0.6	2.1
Figs, dried	30	2 small	0.9	3.0
Flour, all-purpose, enriched	15	2 tablespoons	0.4	2.9
Flour, whole wheat	15	2 tablespoons	0.5	3.3
Hazelnuts	15	10-12	0.6	4.1
Kale	75	¾ cup	1.7	2.2
Lentils, dry	30 (dry)	½ cup (cooked)	2.2	7.4
Molasses, light	20	1 tablespoon	0.9	4.3
Oatmeal	15 (dry)	½ cup (cooked)	0.7	4.5
Parsley	10	10 small sprigs	0.4	4.3
Peaches, dried	30	3 halves	1.9	6.9
Peas, dry	30 (dry)	½ cup (cooked)	1.4	4.7
Pecans	15	12 halves	0.4	2.4

Popcorn	15	1 cup, popped	0.4	2.7
Prunes, dried	30	4 prunes	1.2	3.9
Raisins, dried	50	5 tablespoons	1.7	3.3
Rice, brown	15 (dry)	½ cup (cooked)	0.3	2.0
Rye, whole meal	15	1 tablespoon	0.6	3.7

* Adapted from Krause and Hunscher, Food, Nutrition and Diet Therapy. W.B. Saunders, 1972.

Iodine. Iodine is concentrated by the thyroid gland and is used in the formation of thyroxine. Certain geographical areas, usually far removed from the sea, may be deficient in iodine and are called "goiter belts." Goiters due to iodine deficiency have virtually disappeared in this country since the supplementation of table salt with iodine. Many fruits and vegetables also contain some iodine. Too much iodine can also act as a goitrogen and may be associated with hyperthyroidism.

Selenium. Selenium has an antioxidant effect in the body. It is found in grains and onions. Selenium is lost from food by washing, cooking in large quantities of water, and lengthy storage.

Aluminum. Aluminum salts are the most abundant mineral salts on the crust of the earth. Aluminum is widely distributed in foods. For this reason, it seems unlikely that a deficiency would develop. Some are concerned with toxicity from aluminum obtained from aluminum cookware. With its abundance in nature, a great concern for the small quantities that can be absorbed from the use of aluminum cookware seems unimportant. Yet, because reports have appeared in the medical literature stating that excessive quantities of aluminum have been found at autopsy in the brains of persons who had organic brain disease and senility, it would seem wise to rotate cookware and use steel, enamel, glass, and iron cookware in succession.

Magnesium. Magnesium is a catalyst for numerous biologic functions, particularly in nerve and muscle physiology. Research has suggested that magnesium may control all growth and differentiation and regulate the rate of all functions.[197] Too much calcium can cause a relative deficiency of magnesium. Too much magnesium, as well as manganese, can produce an encephalitis-like condition.

Magnesium is found in bananas, whole grain cereals, dry beans, nuts, peanuts, peanut butter, and most dark, green, leafy vegetables. Grains, legumes, and nuts provide the richest dietary source of magnesium.

Phosphorus. Phosphorus, essential to development of growth and teeth, is found in whole grain cereals, dry beans, peanuts, and peanut butter.

Zinc. In animals, zinc deficiency is characterized by retarded growth, loss of appetite, skin disease, reproductive problems, and poor wound healing. Many of the same characteristics, as well as accelerated atherosclerosis, are now being described in humans who are zinc deficient. Zinc and pyridoxine deficiency can result in spotted fingernails. Bending of the nails may result from hormonal changes during the menstrual cycle and may have to do with fluctuations of minerals under the influence of changing hormone levels. The copper level in the blood is high and zinc levels low about one week before the menstrual period. The minimum daily requirement for zinc is 15 mg, and a deficiency can be aggravated by excess copper, estrogen therapy, and increased iron intake. A diet high in calcium or phytates (as in whole grains and beans) could predispose to zinc deficiency. In diabetes, a zinc deficiency should be carefully avoided. Zinc is a constituent of the hormone insulin.

Long-term vegetarian women do not have reduction in serum iron or zinc, despite their avoidance of flesh foods which have apparently a more readily absorbed form of both iron and zinc. To determine the iron and zinc status of people taking a vegetarian diet, 56 Seventh-day Adventist women were investigated using hemoglobin, serum iron, total iron binding capacity, and serum and hair zinc concentrations. All levels were within normal range. The increased intake of phytates in these women did not cause them to have reduced levels of the minerals usually believed to be significantly bound by phytates.[198]

In prostate disorders, zinc has been found to be beneficial. It is present in all natural foods, especially peas, carrots, whole grains, wheat germ, and sunflower seeds, but is not high in fruits, vegetables, or refined foods. Of course, the malabsorption syndromes may cause zinc deficiency. Similarly, hemodialysis may produce zinc deficiency. There is no indication that psychiatric stress affects zinc nutrition, although it is known that the brains of some chronic schizophrenic patients show abnormally low concentrations of zinc in the hippocampus. The availability of zinc in wheat is increased in leavened breads, which may be due to the longer cooking that occurs when leavening is used. Grains need long, slow cooking. For whole grains used for porridge, mush, or entire grain dishes, the cooking time should be over an hour at boiling temperatures.

Zinc Content of Common Foods[199]

Food	mg/100 gm (edible portion)
Beef, separable lean, cooked, dry heat	5.8
Beans, common, mature, dry	2.8
Beans, lima	2.8
Breads	
Rye	1.6
White	0.6
Whole wheat	1.8
Chickpeas or garbanzos	2.7
Corn, field, whole grain, white or yellow	2.1
Corn, sweet, yellow	0.5
Corn meal, white or yellow, bolted (nearly whole grain)	1.8
Cowpeas (black eyed), mature	2.9
Granola	2.1
Lentils, mature	3.1
Oatmeal (rolled oats)	3.4
Oat cereal, puffed, ready-to-eat	3.0
Peanuts, raw	2.9
Peanuts, roasted	3.0
Peanut butter	2.9
Peas	3.2
Popcorn	4.1
Rice, brown	1.8
Whole wheat	3.4
Wheat germ	14.3
Wheat (shredded wheat)	2.8

Trace Elements. The essential trace elements can be defined as those necessary in less than 100 milligram amounts daily. Milligram quantities of iron, zinc, magnesium, and manganese are described, but microgram quantities are used to describe the daily intake of selenium, chromium, and vanadium. A microgram is 1/1000 of a milligram. Twenty-five to thirty grams of all trace elements (about one ounce) exist in the human body. By contrast, over 1000 grams of calcium exist in the human body. "Lack of certain minerals may be the single most important factor causing a chronic fatigue in conditioned athletes.... The only way to guarantee adequate trace elements in the diet is to eat a wide variety of fruits, vegetables, grains, and nuts," according to Dr. Gabe Mirkin of Silver Springs, Maryland. The diet must be varied because we cannot expect all fruits and vegetables to contain similar amounts of minerals; and also, plants grown in soil deficient in trace elements produce fruits and vegetables with similar deficiencies.[200]

CHAPTER TEN

Condiments, Additives, and Herbs

Stimulating and Sedating Foods

Many foods are made more palatable by the addition of some seasonings. While palatability is the main purpose of adding herbs and other flavorings, traces of minerals are thereby added that may be difficult to obtain from any other source than the flavoring. It is well known in medicine that certain foods are stimulating and certain are sedative. Spices, refined nutrients of all major categories (carbohydrates, fats, minerals, vitamins, and proteins), vinegar, caffeine, etc., are stimulatory, while bland foods, fruits, and vegetables are all sedating; alcohols are depressing. Vitamin and mineral supplements are generally stimulating, and it is this quality that makes a person feel a benefit is being derived from the supplements. Especially during the first few weeks after beginning a course of supplementation, one may feel very good. Vitamin B-12 shots are especially noted for this feature. The effect, however, is no recommendation for the supplement, any more than for the stimulation from caffeine drinks. When the stimulus to the metabolism wears off, the person feels worse than before, and often begins to study what new supplement may be taken to achieve a sense of well being again. Another answer for feeling good should be sought from the beginning--perhaps more exercise or sleep, less food, a program of regularity, or some other adjustment in lifestyle is needed. To eat fast is stimulatory (to digestion and to appetite). While not all stimulatory foods are harmful, generally the stimulatory foods are more likely to be harmful than are calming foods. Some foods or food derivatives first stimulate, then depress or burden the system. Fats fall in this category as do certain preservatives, also theobromine from chocolate and theophyllin from pekoe tea.

Per capita consumption of mayonnaise, salad dressing, and related products went from an annual three pints in 1941 to nine pints in 1971. These foods contain stimulating factors such as oil, vinegar, eggs, salt, sugar, spices, and preservatives. Some types of pickles can cause marked changes in the human stomach, possibly leading to stomach cancer. Population groups using more pickles, soy sauce, vinegar, and heavily salted foods are also more likely to have stomach cancer. Among the condiments can be included salt, pepper, and commercial sauces which contain large proportions of these two seasonings. Cayenne pepper is stimulatory to the nervous system.

Spices

Spices are usually defined as parts, generally bark, seeds, or fruit, of plants having a tropical origin. Herbs come from the leafy parts of temperate zone plants. Cinnamon, ginger, cloves, allspice, mace, anise seed, caraway, celery seed, chili powder, curry powder, mustard, cayenne pepper, hot paprika, and poppy seed are all listed as spices. These substances have varying quantities of irritating chemicals in them necessitating care in their use. Black pepper has been implicated as hazardous to the health. Mice exposed to an extract of black pepper applied to the skin for a long time developed more lung, liver and skin cancers. All three forms of pepper (red, black, and white) have been shown to cause focal areas of necrosis and hemorrhage in the stomach. Black pepper contains a substance that may be cancer producing.[201] It has been determined by scientists at the University of Texas that black pepper and certain other spices, notably turmeric, alter cells permanently. Turmeric causes breaks in chromosomes in such a way as to alter the normal cell's ability to reproduce itself. Such as alteration could lead to cancer, or to deformities in offspring.

Allergies to various spices have been reported. As with any food, should an allergy occur, the person should refrain from using that food, not just to avoid discomfort, but because the unpleasant symptoms of the allergy may be the signal that other organ systems are also being damaged.

There is good evidence to show that certain spices are especially damaging to the kidneys, causing damage to the tubules, producing stones, etc. The countries where there is a high incidence of kidney stone include parts of India and Mexico where curry and other hot spices are quite popular.[202, 203] Commercial meat sauces are associated with recurrent renal stone formation. Damage to the kidney tubules, with excessive excretion of amino acids, may be responsible. The volatile oils in the spices of the commercial meat sauces are toxic to the kidney (nephrotoxic).

There are various condiments and spices that contain acids or volatile oils potentially harmful to the kidney. These include vinegar, garlic, black pepper, ginger, allspice, mace and cinnamon. Worchestershire sauce, which contains certain spices, may be damaging to the kidney.[204] The first symptom may be a sensation of not feeling well, or having blood in the urine, or loss of appetite. Spices may also severely irritate the urinary bladder. Any person subject to cystitis should entirely avoid spices, as well as other foods commonly causing food sensitivities.

Monosodium Glutamate

Monosodium glutamate is a white powder derived from vegetable protein which enhances the flavor of foods rather than representing a flavor of its own. In high dosage, it has been reported to cause brain damage in a variety of young animals. Acute toxic symptoms that are reversible can occur in adults, the so-called Chinese restaurant syndrome. In the body monosodium glutamate degrades to sodium and glutamic acid, an amino acid. Authorities seem to be divided on the safety of this substance;[205,206] it seems clear that it should not be used in *any* amount by infants. If used by adults, it should be in very small quantities until its safety and toxic properties are further clarified.

Chromosome Breakage

In 1949, Kilhman and Levan demonstrated that caffeine causes chromosomal alterations in plants. These chromosomal alterations in plants and animals are termed *mutagenic*; that is, capable of producing permanent genetic alterations in cells. Many food additives, edible fats, insecticides, and drugs are also mutagenic. Ginger has been studied for its mutagenic effects. Ginger contains oleoresin, gingerin, and an essential oil which gives the typical aroma of ginger.

Preservatives such as BHT and BHA which are added to dry cereals, potato chips, etc., also cause damage to chromosomes. Asafetida, cyclamates, and saccharine have been found to be mutagenic and carcinogenic. Certain citrus oils located in the rind, when used in large quantities are cancer-producing ; orange oil and limonene have been tested. Turpentine oil and eucalyptus oil both promote the formation of tumors. Prolonged exposure to even minute quantities of carcinogens may result, after a long latent period, into the development of cancers in exposed individuals.

Other Effects

Some dietary spices and condiments produce hypertension in animals. These include pepper, mustard, and ginger. Eugenol, found in many spices and condiments, can break the mucus barrier of the stomach. Myristicin, in nutmeg, is known to be depressive to the central nervous system.

Spices cause unnatural cravings, unhealthy blood, a desire for too much liquid with meals, irritation of the stomach, and central nervous system irritability. Because of their effect on the central nervous system, spices tend to deaden moral sensibilities.[207, 208, 209, 210, 211, 212]

Gastrointestinal irritation followed by multiple systemic changes is produced by capsicum (cayenne, the hot red peppers). Capsicum has been shown to produce a very large flow of saliva, both in dogs and man. There is a slight increase in mucus secretion in the stomach. It increases intestinal motility slightly, and induces mild diarrhea. Hyperemia (increased blood flow) of the skin occurs following external application of capsicum. When hot peppers, including capsicum, are taken into the stomach, there is an increase in the cutaneous circulation in the abdominal region. The circulation to the hand is not affected, but the circulation to the forehead is diminished in many subjects. These reflexes are termed "viscerocutaneous" and are activated by irritation from capsicum and other hot peppers.[213] A significant increase in stomach acids occurs after ingestion of even minute amounts of red pepper, especially in duodenal ulcer patients.[214]

Essential oils of spices are defined as odorous substances, soluble in alcohol, having limited solubility in water. They are a mixture of esters, aldehydes, ketones, and terpines. Safrol, an odorous substance, is found in anise oil, camphor oil, and especially in sassafras oil. It occurs also in mace, nutmeg, ginger, and cinnamon leaf oil. Safrol was used widely to flavor foods, notably root beer, until it was discovered to cause hepatic adenomas in rats.

Vinegar

Virtually all vinegar sold for food purposes is composed of waste products from bacterial decomposition of apples. Therefore, most vinegar is apple cider vinegar, and one brand is not better than another. The principal chemical giving the sour flavor is acetic acid. This acid, a waste product in the human body, is an irritant to both the stomach and nerves. It is one of the three commonest dietary causes of gastritis in the United States today, along with aspirin and alcohol. All products made with vinegar can just as easily be made with lemon juice, a heathful article. Pickles made with vinegar are injurious to the stomach lining, causing loss of the protective mucus and changes in the lining cells (nuclear enlargement and coarsening of the chromatin and increased mitosis).[216]

Baking Soda

Baking soda leaves residues of injurious salts. Baking powder is baking soda which has been neutralized by the addition of aluminum salts and other compounds which are themselves injurious. Aluminum influence on bean seedlings caused an inhibition of growth in concentrations greater than M/65,536.

In a study by Drs. House and Gies, aluminum was concluded to be toxic to growing cells. When dogs ingested biscuits baked with baking powder, aluminum salts promptly passed into the blood in large amounts. Aluminum occurs in a soluble form in the gastrointestinal tract and is absorbed into the blood. The more thoroughly the bread was baked, the less aluminum passed into the blood.

The aluminum is carried by the blood to all cells of the body. In Alzheimer's disease, severe degeneration of brain tissue, aluminum is concentrated in portions of the brain. Aluminum is used by the body in only minute amounts, and even when a small excess shows up in the urine, it implies a decided physiologic repugnance. We believe that nothing resembling baking soda should be introduced into the stomach.

Testing the effect of baking powder on living cells revealed that the aluminum influence on bean seedlings caused an inhibition of growth in concentrations greater than m/65,536 (i. e., per liter the molecular weight in grams divided by 65,536). It is a very easy thing to bake breads using either yeast as a leavening agent or using no leavening agent at all. The use of aluminum and sodium leavening products in baking is unneeded and unwise.[217]

One way to reduce excess aluminum in the blood may be to eat plenty of high phosphorus foods. Aluminum and phosphorus in blood serum have been shown to have an inverse relationship with each other; as one goes up, the other goes down.[218]

Eating Between Meals

Eating between meals is not a good practice since it causes retention of food in the stomach longer than is desirable. Fermentation is the result of stagnation of food in the stomach. The irritating products which accumulate with fermentation are a common cause of gastritis. Children who take juices, cookies, and candy between meals appear to be more prone to infection than those who do not.[219]

Other Food Additives

Polysorbate 60, 65, and 80, used as emulsifiers in baked goods and frozen desserts, are synthetic carbohydrates, and their handling may tax human metabolic systems. Sorbitol, obtained from fruits and berries, is about half as sweet as sugar. Since it is more slowly absorbed than sugar, it is therefore believed to be slightly safer for diabetics.

Vanillan is a synthetic version of the main flavor in the vanilla bean. It appears to be safe, but it needs more testing before we can endorse it with complete assurance.[220]

Most foods are safer and more nutritious if prepared at home. Bread is easy to make but requires some time. There is an advantage in baking many loaves at one time, as bread can be stored easily either by freezing or drying into zwieback (melba toast). With home-baked bread, many chemicals can be avoided. The following chemicals, used in commercial bread making, are more or less undesirable: ammonium sulfate and ammonium chloride, used to aid in the fermentation of the dough; sodium chloride to give an even texture to bread; chlorine as a bleach used to increase the whiteness of flour; monocalcium and ammonium bicarbonate as leavening agents; acetic acid and lactic acid as bread preservatives; and flavoring agents such as ethyl formate for a rum flavor, butyric acid for a butter flavor, cinnamaldehyde for a cinnamon flavor, and amylalcohol for a whiskey flavor.[221]

Until recently, almost every processed food with a reddish, brownish color, including canned fruits, gelatins, candy bars, salad dressings, cereals, frankfurters, ice cream, cake mixes, and a variety of drugs and cosmetics contained the synthetic Red II dye. Recently Red II dye was banned, but not until it had had years to cause an increased risk for many diseases, including many cases of hyperactivity in children and restlessness in adults.

Many additives, such as Red II dye, have been used for years and considered safe, just as large amounts of sugar and salt once were. In the same fashion vitamin and mineral preparations are now being used in megadose quantities, which are currently being found to be harmful. Our population is unwittingly exposed to these injurious chemicals, sometimes even writing their damage on the genetic material of humanity. Our race is then marked for all future time, before the dangers are recognized and the material banned. Red II dye, an azo dye derived from naphthalene and known generally as Amaranth, has been shown to increase the number of malignant growths in a variety of tissues. The parent substance of azo dyes is azokazene, a reduction product of nitrobenzene, a synthetic substance not native to the human body.

Dr. Stephen Lackey, Sr., of Lancaster, Pennsylvania, states that the azo dye tartrazine, known commonly as FD&C yellow No. 5 and present in yellow United States certified food color, used in coatings of pharmaceuticals and in many foods, may be the cause of allergic responses in many cases of sensitivity, rather than the specific food or drug.

Health food enthusiasts are not the only persons knowledgeable about the dangers of food additives. The National Cancer Institute states that there is a cancer risk due to food additives used as preservatives, and coloring agents. The United States Government Committee on Nutrition declares that "Too much fat, sugar, and salt are linked directly to heart disease and stroke." The United States Senate Subcommittee on Nutrition and Human Needs proclaimed: "Processed foods containing chemicals and refined sugar are being gobbled up by children with resulting poor nutrition and allergies, fatigue and ills."

Potentially Harmful Food Additives

Additives marked with an asterisk should be avoided in the opinion of physicians and registered dieticians. Those without an asterisk are questionable, and safety has not been established.

Chemical Additive	Use in Food	Hazard Factor to Human	Foods Likely to Contain
*BHA (butylated hydroxyanisole) *BHT (butylated hydroxytoluene)	Preservative Coloring	Suspected of liver ailments and cancer May cause allergic reactions Stored in body fat	Fresh pork and pork sausage, steak sauces, vegetable oils, shortenings, crackers, potato chips, dry cereals, cake mixes, frozen pizzas, instant teas, drink powders, punches, breakfast drinks, doughnuts, vegetables (packed with sauces), packaged potatoes, nuts, canned puddings, toaster tarts, dry yeast

Chemical Additive	Use in Food	Hazard Factor to Human	Foods Likely to Contain
*Caffeine	Coloring Flavoring	Stimulant, diuretic, causes nervousness, heart palpitations; may cause heart defects	Coffee, tea, cocoa, cola, soft drinks
EDTA (calcium disodium) Ethylenediamine tetraacetate	Preservative Flavoring Traps metallic impurities produced during food processing	Linked to kidney disorders; cramps, skin rashes, intestinal problems	Mayonnaise, salad dressings, margarine, canned shellfish, beer, condiments, soft drinks, processed fruits and vegetables
Hydroxylated Lecithin (non-hydroxylated lecithin satisfactory)	Binder	Phosphoric acid and choline are toxic in ink and cosmetics May cause skin irritations	Mayonnaise, ice cream, margarine, soup mixes, candy baked goods, artificial flavors
Lactic acid	Preservative	Caustic Used in textile printing, dyeing	Beer, carbonated beverages, frozen desserts, frozen pizzas, processed cheese, gelatin, pudding desserts, olives
Mono- and Diglycerides (usually animal origin unless specified)	Mixes together ingredients Softener Smoothing agent	May cause genetic changes, cancer, birth defects and abnormalities Fattening	Shortening, margarine, peanut butter, broths, bread, pies, dry roasted nuts, vegetables packaged with sauce, cookies, cakes, ravioli
*Monosodium glutamate (MSG)	Flavoring agent	May cause headaches, chilling, sweating, diarrhea, and chest pain; possible genetic damage Removed from baby foods in 1969	Beer, broths, bouillon cubes, processed cheeses, gefilte fish, canned meats, meat tenderizers, packaged seafood, frankfurters, salad dressings, canned soups, frozen pizzas, Chinese food, dry roasted nuts, soup mixes, vegetables packed with sauce, croutons, tomato sauce, bread crumbs, frozen spinach, tomato paste
*Nitrites, sodium	Preservative Coloring Curing	Toxic Overdoses have caused death Combines in the body with other chemicals to form cancer-causing agents	Bacon, frankfurters, sausages, smoked fish, smoked and processed meats such as ham, bologna, pastrami, salami, tongue, corned beef, frozen pizzas, baby foods
Propyl gallate	Preservative	May damage liver May cause birth defects	Meat products, potato sticks, vegetables packed with sauces, vegetable shortenings and oils, chewing gum, pickles

Chemical Additive	Use in Food	Hazard Factor to Human	Foods Likely to Contain
*Propylene glycol alginate	Thickener Stabilizer	Glycol used as auto antifreeze Other components used as solvent for oils, waxes and lubricants	Cream cheese, ice cream, yogurt, cheese spreads, jelly, frozen desserts, whipped toppings, candies, flavor extracts, beer, salad dressings, soft drinks, mustard, potato chips, crackers
*Red dyes (some, including Allura Red AC)	Coloring	Possibly causes birth defects Cancer suspect	Frankfurters, red gelatin desserts, red candies, soft drinks, red pistachio nuts, red chewing gums, cereals, baked goods
*Saccharin	Inexpensive sugar substitute Diabetic use Non-caloric	Causes allergic response and toxic reactions affecting skin, heart, and gastrointestinal tract Possible cause of tumors and bladder cancer	Sugar substitute in many products and diet foods, ginger ale, plain and diet sodas, frozen desserts, breakfast drinks
*Sodium erythrobate	Preservative Coloring agent Freshening	Possible genetic effects Banned in several countries	Bacon, ham, frozen turkey roast, frankfurters, baked goods, potato salads, beverages
Tannin (tannic acid)	Flavoring	May cause liver tumors and ailments, and other cancers Used widely in leather tanning	Wine, coffee, tea, cocoa, beer, artificial flavorings (butter, fruit, caramel, brandy, maple, nut)

Foods Containing Some of The Potentially Harmful Food Additives

Cakes, crackers, pies and doughnuts contain 11 undesirable additives.

Colas, soft drinks, punches, powders contain 9 undesirable additives.

Pizzas (frozen) contain 6 undesirable additives.

Gelatin and pudding desserts contain 6 undesirable additives.

Ice cream and ice milk contain 6 undesirable additives.

Beer contains 6 undesirable additives.

Vegetable sauces contain 5 undesirable additives.

Broths contain 4 undesirable additives.

Salad dressings contain 4 undesirable additives.

"The labels on these food products read more like concoctions for witches' brews than for the processing of wholesome foods for human consumption." [222]

Avoid These Additives

Alcohol
Baking soda and powder
BHA, BHT
Caffeine
EDTA
Hydroxylated Lecithin
Lactic Acid
Monosodium Glutamate (MSG)
Nitrites, Nitrates
Pepper, Black & Red
Propyl gallate
Propylene glycol alginate
Red dyes
Saccharin and other sugar substitutes
Sodium erythorbate
Spices
Tannin
Vinegar
Mono and Diglycerides

Adapted from Harmful Food Additives. Kroft and Houben. Port Washington, New York: Ashley Books, 1981.

Osteoporosis Encouraged

About half the baking powder in this country is made from baking soda with alum added; the other half has a phosphate compound added. Both of these substances--alum and phosphate compounds--cause osteoporosis. The more baking powder products used, the more damaging to the bones.

High levels of protein also cause osteoporosis. Extra protein is added to food by putting textured vegetarian protein (TVP) in soups, stews and casseroles. Bacon-like commercially prepared bits or chips sprinkled on salads or potatoes also add protein to the diet. The extra protein not only acts to thin the bones, but puts a heavier load on the kidneys and liver than foods of lower protein content.

Many cooks have the belief that adding protein to a dish increases its nourishment. The reverse is true, as most Americans are actually intoxicated on protein already; that is, they have eaten so much protein that the toxic effects are found in many organs.

Salt in generous quantities has a demineralizing effect on bones. Fast food (and generally *all*) restaurants use too much salt. The same must be said of many households. Probably the kitchens of South Georgia salt more heavily than most parts of the United States. A large study done in Evans County, Georgia, demonstrated injury to bones, kidneys and blood vessels due to the excessive use of salt.

Sugar is being focused on more and more along with other types of concentrated sweeteners--honey, malt, syrups, molasses, etc.--as a cause of high insulin levels in the blood of both non-diabetics and diabetics. As the pancreas produces more and more insulin and the level rises in the blood, the irritating results begin in heart, kidneys and blood vessels. Too much insulin is defined as any excess over what would be required to barely maintain weight at an ideal level. Figure your ideal level by allowing 100 pounds for your first five feet, then add five pounds per inch thereafter if you are female, and six to seven pounds per inch thereafter if you are male, depending on how muscular you are. Do not overeat, even if you are thin. The excess calories load down your systems with nutrients, accelerate aging, reduce clarity of though and often add unwanted fat.

CHAPTER ELEVEN

Controls of Thirst and Appetite

Water Requirements and Thirst

Palatability of food, hunger, and thirst are all involved in food intake among humans. Three circumstances are known to arouse thirst: deficiency of water, excess of solutes in the body (hyperosmotic state), and the intake of dry food. Dehydration often results in a high pitched or scratchy voice, a sense of fatigue and langor (much in the way that a plant wilts when dehydrated), dizziness, and faintness. Dehydration of a minor degree can cause a craving for food. An increase in salt in the diet can induce water drinking.

An increase in sweating tends to draw water from the tissues, in order to preserve an intact blood volume. Much sweating, however, increases the osmotic character of the blood, and induces drinking. Similar amounts of sucrose or amino acids will not induce as much tendency to drink as will salt.

Water requirements for one day are in the vicinity of 20 milliliters per pound of body weight or 44 milliliters per kilogram per day. That figures out to about 10-12 glasses per day. Since almost half of this water is contained in prepared foods and produced metabolically, we need to drink only 5-6 glasses. If sweating occurs, more would be needed.[223]

Drink, Drink, Drink

Water is a miracle fluid. Its chemical and physical properties are especially suited to be the perfect solvent in the human body. Cells of the body vary from 60-90% water. Brain cells and intestinal cells are particularly well hydrated. In order to think well, one needs optimum water saturation of the neural tissues.

In the course of a day, one loses water from the skin, intestinal tract, lungs, and kidneys. This water must be replaced by drinking. Further, many people dehydrate their tissues by the use of diuretics such as caffeine (found in coffee, tea, chocolate, and colas) and nicotine, which cause unnatural elimination of water by the kidneys. While these beverages supply some water, the overall effect is one of dehydration because of the diuretic effect on the kidneys.

Can one depend on thirst as a sufficient indication of how much water to drink? Actually thirst is inadequate to promote sufficient drinking, as conversely, appetite in most people is too great to maintain perfect weight. A useful gauge in the matter of drinking water is the color of the urine. Proper hydration will make the urine almost colorless, unless one is taking vitamin supplements, making it impossible to entirely clear the urine. A careful check on this matter and proper corrections should lead one to rarely produce a highly colored urine specimen.

If you do not like tap water, you may find the large bottles of commercial drinking water more palatable. Whether or nor there are other benefits in the use of bottled water has not yet been established scientifically, and probably depends substantially on the type of water purchased. Distilled water and herb teas may also be used to make water drinking more acceptable.

When Shall I Drink Fluids?

It is important that water be taken at the proper time. Upon rising in the morning is a very good time to take water, as it promotes good urine production, an activity which may have been reduced during the night. Further, drinking acts for many as a stimulant to the intestinal tract to initiate emptying.

The latter function may be promoted more by hot than by cold water.

Since fourth grade health classes, most Americans have heard, "Don't wash your food down with fluids." Very few people, however, really understand what this statement means. Water taken with meals cuts down on the production of saliva and discourages chewing, making the length of time food spends in the mouth much shorter. Digestion is thereby hindered. Also, since digestive enzymes both in the mouth and in the stomach and intestines are diluted by beverages taken with meals, digestion is further delayed. The stomach must make more acid to maintain a proper pH. All these factors add to the likelihood of fermentation in the digestive tract, gas formation, and various types of discomfort and poor functioning of digestion and elimination. The lack of understanding people have on this subject probably stems from an inconsistency in the teaching in the classroom and the practice in the lunchroom. After hearing a lecture on not washing food down, the student is sent to lunch where he is served his lunch with juices, punch, or milk. Of course, every place setting includes a glass of water or tea, and his teachers are liberally furnished with coffee. These customs certainly do not illustrate the principles presented by the health teacher.

When should one drink beverages? Never should solid foods, milk, or juices be taken between meals. A good rule is to drink large quantities of water some time before or after meals, preferably thirty minutes or more from mealtime. Except for small quantities, juices, milks, and broths should be taken when one is not eating solid food, such as when one is skipping a meal or trying to fight off a cold. Liquid foods may be taken as a light meal in-stead of a supper of solid foods. The latter is a very good practice, as all digestion should be completed and the stomach empty before one retires for the night.

Controls of Hunger and Appetite

The hypothalamus has been largely assigned the responsibility for regulation of intake of food and water. More specifically, this function has been ascribed to the amygdaloid complex in the brain. The amygdala enhances rather than controls the intake of food and water. At least three conditions are known to affect animal hunger:

1. The degree of starvation (the length of time since the last meal or the percentage of loss in body weight).

2. Factors influencing the rate of energy output, such as metabolic work rate, work level, and environmental temperature (cold temperatures stimulating greater eating than hot temperatures).

3. Rate of energy input in caloric content of the diet, and the nature of the dietary components.

Appetite is different from hunger. It is a complicated psychological activity and depends on a variety of complex, interrelated factors. Four groups of determinants are known to influence the appetite:

1. Constitutional factors, such as disease.

2. Internal conditions produced by deprivation, general health, surgery, the work of the nervous system, etc.

3. Environmental conditions.

4. Psychological factors, acquired dispositions, habits, etc.

CHAPTER TWELVE

Digestion

Functions of the Digestive Tract

The digestion of food is the primary method of obtaining energy for all of the cellular functions of the body. The digestive tract includes the digestive canal, itself, with its associated exocrine and endocrine functions and its appendage organs, especially the liver, biliary tree, and pancreas. The functions of the digestive tract are as follows:

1. the receipt of food.
2. The mechanical and chemical breakdown of food.
3. The transport of materials along the tube.
4. The absorption of all nutritious portions.
5. Discharge of waste products.
6. Excretion of toxic substances from the blood.
7. Ancillary functions such as antibody production, water balance, etc.

Acid, mucus, enzymes, hormones, bile, and other factors are produced to assist in these functions.

Mouth

The mouth has certain structures peculiarly adapted to its functions:

Teeth. The teeth are a masterpiece of engineering genius. They are stable, yet not cemented in position. This feature greatly reduces the likelihood of cracking, as they have some give at the sockets. Teeth are comprised of enamel, the hardest material in the human body, dentin, nerves, and blood vessels. Interestingly, they possess a tubular network that functions as a circulatory system throughout the enamel, dentin, and pulp. There are incisors for cutting, and molars for grinding.

Tongue. The tongue is a muscular organ covered with taste buds which have four possible sensations: salt, sour, bitter, and sweet. By combining and varying the intensity of the various sensations, a number of other tastes, such as metallic, electric, and alcoholic can be appreciated. The tongue propels food backward through a complex series of muscular contortions. The tongue is also capable of the most fine muscular movements of any muscle group of the body, being able to maneuver a tiny seed between two teeth, a feat the fingers would find impossible.

The Salivary Glands. The parotid glands are located just in front of and below the ear and around the angle of the mandible. They are most commonly affected by the mumps virus. The submaxillary glands are located in the fleshy part of the floor of the mouth. The sublingual glands are located under the tongue. The duct which discharges saliva from each of these three major groups of salivary glands can be identified in the mouth with a hand mirror. Wipe the surface dry and watch for a minute or two until a small droplet of saliva appears at the opening of the duct. Some one and one-half quarts of saliva are produced each day; this includes the saliva produced during ordinary maintenance and during the digestion of food. Saliva is not produced at a uniform rate at all times, but is especially abundant during chewing and digestion. However, it is scanty during periods of stress, fear, and anxiety. The mucus in saliva is very small in amount, but because of its slipperiness, extremely useful. Ten times as much saliva would be needed just to get the food masticated and swallowed if there were no mucus in the saliva!

The Esophagus

The esophagus is a tube which has the duty of transporting the chewed food from the mouth to the stomach. At the upper end, there are numerous muscles which compress and propel the ball of food downward to the lower one-third of the esophagus. There the food may rest until two or three other balls of food join the first one before the cardia opens.

The cardia is a muscular thickening that guards the opening between the esophagus and the stomach, preventing reflux of material from the stomach into the esophagus. It is at this point in the digestive tract that a hiatus hernia may occur. The hiatus hernia is a protrusion upward of a portion of the stomach into the chest where only the lower portion of the esophagus should be. It is caused by increased intra-abdominable pressure, such as may be caused by overweight, constipation with straining at the stool, and the wearing of tight bands (such as girdles and belts) around the abdomen. Esophageal reflux without hiatus hernia occurs when the gastroesophageal sphincter is paralyzed by such things as drugs, overeating, caffeine, nicotine, eating between meals, and eating before bedtime. The symptoms of heartburn, esophagitis, difficulty in swallowing, and choking are essentially the same as for hiatus hernia.

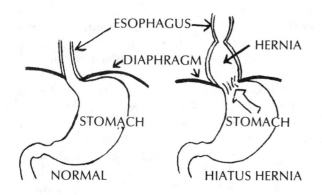

The normal esophagus and the mechanism of a hiatus hernia. The diaphragm muscle stretches across the midpoint of the abdomen and the chest cavity. The hernia occurs at the juncture of the stomach and the esophagus as a result of weakness or relaxation of the opening in the diaphragm.

Stomach

The stomach is a tubular organ no larger in diameter than the colon when collapsed. However, when filled, it can hold two quarts or more of

material. The top part of this muscular organ is called the fundus; the mid-portion, the body; and the lower end, the bulb, which ends in the pylorus. An air bubble often collects in the fundus due to swallowed air. This bubble causes much discomfort for babies after nursing.

A muscular sphincter, called the pylorus, guards the lower opening. It allows only a small bit of chyme (the mixture of food, saliva, and gastric juices) from the stomach to pass through into the duodenum only on certain signals which indicate the duodenum is ready to receive it. Peristaltic waves begin at the top of the stomach and move downward over the stomach in a napkin ring fashion to end at the pylorus. The peristaltic waves pass successively over the stomach until finally one strong wave passes on into the pylorus, opening it and dilating the duodenum a small amount. With the strong pylorus-opening wave, a small amount of acid chyme from the stomach is squeezed into the duodenum.

Each day, 2 to 2.5 quarts of gastric juice are produced. The stomach maintains a pH of 1.5 to 3.0. The major digestants secreted by the stomach are hydrochloric acid and pepsin. Other enzymes and mucus are also produced there. The emptying time of the stomach is one to four hours, depending on the food eaten. Carbohydrates empty most rapidly, protein next, and fats slowest at ten grams (approximately two teaspoons) per hour.

Carbohydrate is sometimes abnormally dumped from the stomach into the duodenum; ignoring the signals or perhaps never receiving them. Then the blood sugar level rises too quickly and too high, as do other nutrients, to activate a rebound disorder described elsewhere as reactive hypoglycemia.

Rice boiled soft in water will empty from the stomach at a rate of about two hours and forty minutes for 100 grams (almost ⅓ cup). If milk and sugar are added to the rice before cooking, the 100 grams require three hours and thirty minutes to get through the stomach, indicating the greater toll exacted by the more concentrated foods from the stomach. Milk-sugar combinations require a longer processing time. This allows greater opportunity for fermentation. Also, milk causes the stomach to produce more acid than do cereals.[224]

Duodenum

The duodenum is the first portion of the gastrointestinal tract concerned with significant assimilation of nutrients into the blood. This absorption of nutrients is accomplished by a fine network of blood capillaries in the intestinal wall which take up the nutrients from the digested material and take them to the liver for processing. The secretion of the duodenum is alkaline. It contains duodenal juice, bile, and pancreatic secretions.

The duodenum begins receiving food within a few minutes after food is eaten if the person is very hungry. If there is no hunger, the meal may not be delivered to the duodenum for two to three hours after the food is eaten. The material from the stomach is propelled along the duodenum and jejunum at a fairly brisk pace. Yet, the chemical reactions that break down food substances into the elementary particles have barely enough time to get completed. In this portion of the small bowel, with 90% of assimilation going on in the first ten inches, a veritable chemical explosion occurs. Still, the production of heat is not excessive, the pH is not seriously altered, and the hemostasis in the duodenum is maintained fairly well. The Divine Chemist arranged digestion very well. No part of digestion is in process of evolving. It is complete.

Both the secretions from the pancreas and those from the liver are alkaline, making the duodenum quite alkaline in contrast to the stomach which is quite acid.

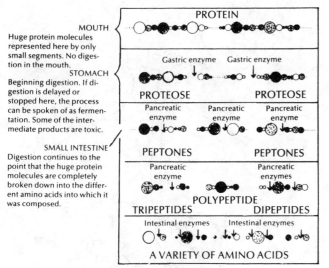

Adapted from Bogert, Briggs, & Calloway, NUTRITION AND PHYSICAL FITNESS, 9th ed. W.B. Saunders, 1973, p. 312.

Small Intestine

The indigestible residue and the 10% of yet-to-be-digested food is propelled along the rest of the jejunum to the ileum. The jejunum and ileum are both classified as small intestine. The ileum contains in its lining aggregates of lymphocytes which apparently have the same function here as in the tonsils and appendix, a function which will be discussed later. A major function of the small intestine is absorption of nutrients. The meshwork of fine blood capillaries which ramify through the lining cells of the intestine are the primary anatomical units for absorption. The work is accomplished by the following mechanisms:

Diffusion. When solutions such as mineral salts, or alcohol and water, which are capable of mixing are placed in separate layers in the same vessel, they will mix slowly by diffusion without stirring. If a crystal of blue copper sulfate is dropped into a glass of water and left for several days, the entire glass of water will turn a uniform blue color. This dispersion of the color is accomplished by diffusion. No energy is required to effect diffusion from the intestinal contents through the lining cells.

Osmosis. Small molecules dissolved on one side of a semipermeable membrane separating two compartments of fluids will cross to the other side to form an equilibrium, resulting in the same concentration of molecules on each side of the membrane. Fluid may transfer if the solid particles cannot cross the membrane. In either event, the end result is equalization of the concentration of fluid and solid particles on both sides of the membrane. No energy is required for this type of transfer of materials.

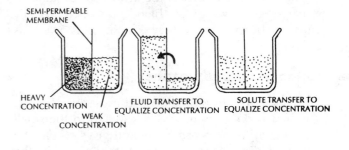

Carrier Systems. In this method of transfer, an agent must carry a large, fat-soluble or other substance "piggyback" across the cell membrane. An example of this is vitamin B-12 which apparently must be carried by intrinsic factor. By some mechanisms, which we do not fully understand, one substance attaches or dissolves a second substance which is the essential nutrient to be delivered inside the cell, the carrier substance itself being used in the process also. Sugar and amino acids have specific carriers. Some carrier mechanisms require energy to operate them, in contrast to the first two mechanisms listed.

Pores. These are openings in the lipoprotein of the cell membrane to allow water-soluble molecules to enter. The transfer of materials is by diffusion, with no work required.

Pumps. While simple diffusion and osmosis require no work, the pumps, since they must operate uphill against the gradient of concentration, require a considerable expenditure of energy. The known pumps include the sodium pump, the glucose pump, and the calcium pump. Additionally, the absorption of sodium, glucose, amino acids, calcium, iron, and B-12 requires both carriers and a pump.

Pinocytosis. This is a sort of "drinking" by the cell. It is probably not a normal way to absorb nutrients and may result in whole, undigested proteins being absorbed at times. Homogenization of milk is said to favor the absorption of whole proteins of milk, perhaps by this process. The immature digestive tract of the infant who is formula-fed or given solid foods too early may absorb whole proteins or large parts of protein molecules by this method. It is believed by many that absorption of unprepared protein in this way can set the stage for allergies in later life. In a Belgian report, 46 newborns who had received dairy milk were studied. In every case, immune complexes containing entire bovine milk proteins were found in the children's blood serum. The researchers expressed concern, since large immune complexes are known to be able to damage the lining of blood vessels, possibly causing heart and kidney damage, as well as allergies.[225]

Colon or Large Intestine

The large intestine is divided into several parts. The first is the cecum, which is joined to the small intestine at the ileocecal valve and gives rise to the appendix. The second part of the colon is the ascending colon. Next comes the hepatic flexure, then the transverse colon, the splenic flexure, the descending colon, the sigmoid, and the rectum. The rectum is closed by the anus.

The appendix has an important function and should not be removed surgically except for life-threatening disorders. The appendix is one of the important lymphoid aggregates in the body. It is ideally situated to sense bacterial secretions and to produce antibodies against these antigens. The

tubular structure of the appendix allows germs from the colon to enter the appendix, where the germs are exposed at close range to the lymphocytes which line the appendix. The lymphocytes "sense" the nature of the germs, which act as antigens, and produce antibodies against the germs. This activity of the appendix helps to augment the total immune armament of the body. Those in the population who have lost the appendix for any reason are at a slightly, but significantly, increased risk of cancer within the abdomen. The appendix should not be needlessly removed during another surgical procedure.

The remainder of the colon is for storage and for absorbing water and vitamins some of which are made in the colon, others having escaped absorption up the line. Bacteria can break down any digestible food residue to make aldehydes, amines, hydrogen, carbon dioxide, etc., which are absorbed into the blood stream and can be detected in the exhaled breath. Some of the substances are toxic, initially, while others combine with other food fragments to become toxic. It seems proper to postulate that any bacterial action on digestible residues of food is undesirable because of discomfort and potential injury from the by-products.

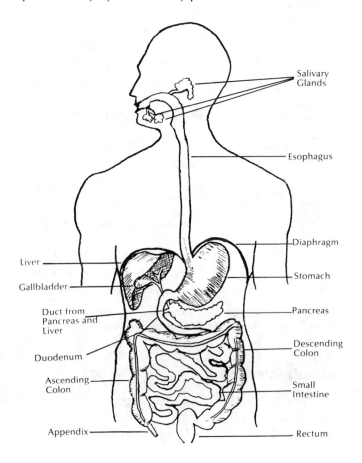

Liver and Gallbladder

The liver is the largest gland of the body and performs vital functions that cannot be taken over by any other part of the body. It produces, among other things, bile which is stored and concentrated in the gallbladder. The bile contains water, bile salts, bile acids, cholesterol, lecithin, and mucus. The gallbladder empties on signal from *secretin* and *cholecystokinin*, hormones from the duodenum. One of the major functions of bile is to emulsify fats so they can be acted upon by digestive enzymes and absorbed.

Major Functions of the Liver

1. To help accomplish the metabolism of protein, carbohydrate, and lipids.
2. Conjugation and detoxification of various toxic substances (such as excess hormones and food fragments which occur as intermediary products during the digestion of food) produced in the body, and foreign substances from outside the body, such as drugs, food, and inhalants.
3. Synthesis of proteins in cooperation with the pancreas.
4. The maintenance of a proper blood sugar level in cooperation with the pancreas.
5. Formation of many precursor substances to be used in the manufacturing processes of a wide variety of other tissues and cells.

Major Functions of the Pancreas

There are two major functions of the pancreas. The endocrine portion puts two hormones directly into the blood stream without employing a system of ducts, the hormones diffusing into the blood; and the exocrine which performs the function of delivering enzymes the pancreas produces to the duodenum by means of a duct system. Insulin is one of the two hormones the endocrine system of the pancreas produces. Both sugar and amino acids are increased in production in the body and released for use through the action of insulin on the liver. Insulin enables the cells to take up the sugar from the blood and utilize it for energy or fat production. Without insulin, the cellular energy cycle is interrupted, and the person gradually starves to death. Insulin also lowers the blood sugar after a meal, preventing the blood from becoming syrupy. Glucagon, the second of the secreted hormones, has many functions. One of these functions is to prevent the blood sugar from going too low. In some ways it balances and complements the funtion of insulin.

The exocrine function involves that of production of trypsin, amylase, and lipase. These enzymes digest the major energy nutrients, protein, carbohydrates, and fats respectively. Their production is controlled by a time signal as well as by chemical signs from secretin, a hormone made in the duodenum.

General Principles of Digestion

Any defect in one phase of digestion hampers another. As an example: Eating between meals not only increases stomach emptying time, but also confuses the colon so that defecation schedule may be altered, resulting in constipation. Certain substances may be absorbed without any digestion; these are water, monosaccharides (glucose, etc.), and inorganic ions. The lipids, di—and poly-saccharides, and proteins must be broken down into more simple constituents before they can be absorbed. It can be readily ascertained that there is no advantage in eating meat, since the meat must be broken down into its individual units before it can be absorbed by the small intestine. It is just as well to get the original nutrients firsthand, since ultimately the source of all nutrients is living plants or the soil.

Chewing is essential to proper digestion. To mix saliva with the food is highly desirable. After being swallowed, the mass of food may remain in the fundus of the stomach from one-half to two hours while salivary digestion of the starch continues. The digestive juices will cause the chyme to be approximately 50% water. If additional portions of water or beverages are taken with the meal, especially if ice cold, digestion is greatly retarded. Violent exercise, either mental or physical, immediately after a meal retards digestion. Mild exercise, however, promotes digestion.

Fat Digestion and Absorption

Because a large quantity of fat dumped into the blood stream at one time is deleterious to health and might fatally clog the circulatory system, a mechanism for retardation of stomach emptying of fat is present. When a bit of fat enters the duodenum, a chemical message is sent to the brain which then signals the stomach to cease releasing more material into the duodenum until it has taken care of the fat. Fat may stay in the stomach for four hours or longer, producing at the time a sensation of satiety (filled with food) but rendering fermentation more likely. Since fermentation products irritate the stomach, and an irritated stomach subsequently evokes a greater sensation of hunger, the practice of eating fats for satiety is self-defeating. It truly can be said that fats clog the digestion. Much pain and indigestion have their origin with the fats eaten.

In the small bowel, emulsification with bile first occurs, and then lipase breaks the fat molecules and splits off two of the three fatty acids from triglycerides. The resulting monoglyceride and the two fatty acids are also emulsified by the bile. A cluster of molecules comprised of bile salts, fatty acids, and monosaccharides attach themselves to the cell membranes of the small bowel. The complex enters the cell by dissolving the lipid part of the phospholipid of the cell membrane. Bile salts are then released from their union and re-enter the intestine. Sixty to seventy per cent of fat thus digested is absorbed by means of the lymph vessels. The fat travels up the large lymph vessels by being squeezed by adjacent pressures (backflow being prevented by valves) and is gradually discharged into the blood stream in a large vein in the chest.

Protein Digestion and Absorption

The stomach initiates protein digestion. It is interesting to note that milk is not easy to digest. Milk protein and carbohydrate are best digested by two special digestants—rennin and lactase, respectively. These two powerful enzymes are present in the digestive fluids of babies only. In persons of Northern European stock, 45% do not have this enzyme in adulthood. North Americans are reported to have a lactase deficiency in adults varying in incidence from 16-55%, the higher rates being seen in blacks. The lactose in milk goes over into the colon undigested, in those deficient in lactase, to be acted on by the colon bacteria. Fermentation is the result, with acids and gas produced, resulting in discomfort, mental dullness, headaches, bad breath, and many other symptoms.

Rennin curdles milk in infants. After rennin production is lost, at around two years of age, acid takes over the function of curdling milk but does so less effectively than rennin. The solid curd formed by the action of rennin is in better condition than liquid milk to be acted upon by pepsin, breaking down the molecules of protein into proteoses and peptones. For this reason, milk digestion is a much greater tax on digestion in adults than in babies.

Free hydrochloric acid changes pepsinogen to pepsin, which accomplishes the peptic digestion of protein. About 90% or more of the food in an ordinary mixed diet is digested and assimilated. Trypsin and other proteolytic enzymes from the pancreas continue the digestion of proteins to the simplest amino acids. There is good evidence that it is the absorption of amino acids through the small bowel mucosa that effects the release of insulin from the pancreatic cells. The digestive tract is a very active area. During the digestion of a single meal, about eight quarts of fluid from the body pass back and forth across the lining of the intestinal tract to keep the nutrients in solution and to keep them moving in a proper direction.

When food is absorbed from the intestinal tract, it is carried first to the liver for "inspection" and detoxification, if necessary. It is not generally recognized that many foods carry some toxic properties. The common white potato manufactures the toxic substance solanine. The average content of this alkaloid is about 8 mg per 100 grams of potato. The interior of the potato contains less, the skin more. The toxic dose is 20-25 mg.

A hotel proprietor and his family of four ate potatoes baked in their jackets for supper on three successive Sunday evenings. All who ate the skins were ill on each occasion, with vomiting, diarrhea, and abdominal pain. The onset of symptoms did not occur for eight hours or more after supper, and recovery was complete in every instance. The hotel proprietor, who ate only the flesh of the potatoes each time, remained well. Analysis showed 50 mg of solanine per 100 grams of potatoes; twenty times as high as potatoes purchased locally. Similar alkaloids are also found in tomatoes, peppers, and eggplant. When potatoes have been responsible for poisoning, the potatoes have often shown unusual features: a pink color developing on the cut surfaces, a brownish line near the surface, an acrid taste, or they were sprouting.[226]

Several legumes have toxic properties in the raw state. Kidney beans were used raw in feeding experiments and found to be toxic for rats. They lost weight quickly and died after a short time if as much as 40% of their diet was composed of raw kidney beans.[227] Many people will get a stomach-ache or other toxic symptoms from eating raw legumes or unsteamed sprouts from legumes.

Psychological Factors Influencing Digestion

Attractive, happy surroundings in an atmosphere of gratitude to the Creator increase the efficiency of digestion and assimilation. Negative emotions such as anger, anxiety, and discontent have an inhibitory effect on the functions of secretion and peristalsis. Thoughts affect the hypothalamus, which influences the autonomic nervous system to bring about these inhibitions. A prayer of thanksgiving to God before a meal, however, has a salutary effect on digestion.

Fecal Flora

Many bacteria live as commensals by symbiosis in the gastrointestinal tract. That is, bacteria live together with human hosts, receiving nourishment from a common source. Certain gases are produced in the colon by action of the bacteria on undigested carbohydrate particles and polysaccharides such as cellulose. When gas is produced, it is also quite likely that acid will be produced by the bacteria at the same time. Acids cause irritation and pain. It is the acid that causes most of the discomfort in flatus production, not the distension of the colon. Hydrogen, carbon dioxide, ammonia, methane, and other gases are also produced. Acids such as lactic acid and acetic acid are formed in the colon during degradation of carbohydrates. Various toxic substances such as aldehydes, amines, indole, phenol, and skatole are also produced. Protein or fat degradation by fecal flora yields most of the unpleasant odors of intestinal gas, not carbohydrate decomposition.

CHAPTER THIRTEEN

Metabolism

The Position of Enzymes in Metabolism

Every cell elaborates thousands of enzymes which are required for use in its metabolic processes. These enzymes must all be preformed and ready to go. If there were no other support for divine creation of the universe, the enormous complexity of these cellular enzymes alone would make the theory of evolution impossible to believe. Without them, life is impossible. Cellular enzymes must be passed down from a parent cell in order for growth and development to start in the daughter cell. Reflection on the process, candidly examining all aspects of the matter, must lead one to the conclusion that chance alone could never develop a cell, given any set of ideal circumstances the mind can devise.

Some enzymes, such as pepsin, are almost entirely protein, while others are largely non-protein. The non-protein part is called a coenzyme. Coenzymes are usually small, organic molecules which always contain a phosphate group and nearly always contain B-vitamins. The enzymes and coenzymes speed up the biologic reactions within the cell. Mitochondria are located in the cell and have to do with cellular respiration. Various respiratory enzymes are produced by the mitochondria. The sum total of processes that use or make energy produced by the millions of tiny chemical reactions that occur in various cells throughout the course of a day, both to build up as well as to break down substances, is called metabolism.

One of the main functions of enzymes is to act as organic catalysts. In serving this function, they speed up the rate at which chemical reactions occur. The way this takes place may be explained by the "collision" theory. The velocity of a particle in solution, as well as the molecular geometry of the particle, determines whether any given particle will make contact with another particle to enable a chemical reaction to occur. If a molecule collides with an atom or another molecule in such a way that the portion of the molecule that can react is turned away from the atom or molecule, no reaction can occur. If, however, some device holds the first molecule into position so that the reactive portion is more exposed to colliding atoms or molecules, the reaction will proceed much faster. Enzymes have the ability to hold molecules in position and thereby speed chemical reactions. This is why our bodies can operate at a dynamic steady state at a relatively low temperature and pressure. We get energy at 37 degrees C. and one atmosphere pressure. Most engines burn gas at around 1300 degrees C. and develop thousands of pounds of pressure when the air-gasoline mixture explodes. What a marvelous system the Creator has designed to tap the energy source He designed to operate quietly and smoothly—in flesh!

Basal Metabolism

The basal metabolism rate (BMR) is the rate at which oxygen is utilized in the various metabolic processes when the body is in a state called basal. In this state, the body is awake, but completely relaxed, not digesting food, not under the influence of drugs, and not troubled with any mental, emotional, or physical condition such as fever. A tall, thin person has a greater skin surface compared to body weight than a short, stout person. Therefore, a higher BMR is needed to keep up such functions as heat loss from the surface, and the energy requirements for muscular movements.

Muscle tissue has a higher BMR than either adipose or connective tissue. Women, therefore, have a BMR some 5 to 10% lower than men, because of the greater preponderance of muscle tissue in man. Athletes have a BMR 5% higher than non-athletes. In cases of loss of muscle tissue, such as occurs in starvation, the BMR may be decreased up to 50%. Part of this is the body's normal mechanism for conserving energy during starvation, but part is due to reduced function of tissue having a high BMR.

During sleep, the BMR goes down approximately 10-15% below that of the waking level. In hot climates, the BMR is often reduced by 10-15%. Heavy foods taken in hot weather can work against this natural reduction in the BMR to cause discomfort. "The less sugar introduced into the food in its preparation, the less difficulty will be experienced because of the heat of the climate."[228, 229] The presence of a fever causes the BMR to rise about 7% for each degree Fahrenheit of fever. Part of this rise is accounted for by an elevation in the heart rate, which increases about ten beats per minute for each degree of fever.

Stress increases the basal metabolic rate. A person going through a divorce, a business reversal, or a tragedy of some kind may lose weight on the very same diet as before the event because of the action of stress on the basal metabolic rate. Each additional decade of life costs one approximately 5% reduction in basal metabolic rate after age 25. After age 75, the basal metabolic rate drops approximately 7% per decade. It is necessary, then, that food intake be progressively reduced as each decade passes. This decline accounts for the fact that many people gradually accumulate weight on the same diet they used in youth.

Metabolism and Energy

Metabolism is essentially an expression of energy relationships. Green leaves make energy from the sun available to all other living beings. Animals are unable to manufacture their food directly. The energy stored by plants is available to the animal, provided the animal has the proper enzymes. Wood and coal contain abundant sources of energy, but animals have no enzymes capable of releasing this energy. The energy from the breakdown of foodstuffs is stored in high energy bonds of the adenosine diphosphate and adenosine triphosphate (ADP-ATP) system. This is largely accomplished through the tricarboxylic acid cycle, a common pathway in the metabolism of all three major nutrients: carbohydrates, fats, and proteins. Some of the energy from carbohydrates is used for synthesis of adenosine triphosphate (ATP) in the energy cycle pictured below. The high energy phosphate bond stores energy which it subsequently makes available for cellular metabolism.

If one depends on a high protein diet to supply part of the daily calories, about 15% more food must be added, as a part of the protein molecule cannot be recovered from the energy chain. Proteins yield 58% of their weight as available glucose, fats 10%, but carbohydrates over 95%. Captain Joseph Bates, a sea captain during the 1840's, made certain observations at Liverpool, England, where two Irishmen "were shoveling salt from a scow into his vessel. Seven or eight men were unable to shovel it into the hold of the vessel as fast as these two Irishmen were scooping it to them through the 'ballast port.' In commenting on the situation, he learned that while the crew of the ship were living in good boardinghouses in Liverpool, the Irishmen had eaten no flesh for some time, and were living on vegetables. By this incident he was forcibly impressed with the fact that flesh food does not impart 'superior strength to the laboring class' "[230]

ENERGY CHAIN

Energy + CO_2 + H_2O (SUN)

DIETARY CARBOHYDRATE COMPOSED OF C_1 H_1 O_2

O_2 -PO_4 ATP ATP ~P ADP

-PO_4 AMP ADP

~ P HIGH ENERGY PHOSPHATE BOND

SYNTHESIS (ANABOLISM)   STORAGE (CATABOLISM)

CHAPTER FOURTEEN

Endocrinology

Adrenals

The adrenals are divided into two portions, the cortex (bark) and the medulla (marrow). The adrenal medulla is responsible for producing the hormone adrenalin. The adrenal medulla, being derived from the nervous system, has a different embryologic development from that of the cortex. Because of its embryonic origin, it has very easy communication with the nervous system and can readily respond to thoughts, sights, and sounds.

It is this quality that enables the adrenal to produce adrenalin on a moment's notice in response to shocking events. One sees a frightening sight and adrenalin is discharged within seconds into the blood stream. The pupils dilate, the hair stands on end, the bowel becomes quiet, the saliva gets thick and mucoid, and the blood pressure and pulse rise.

While adrenalin serves an important function, it is not vital to life. The destruction of the adrenal medulla by disease does not result in a life-threatening disorder. The same cannot be said of the adrenal cortex, however. The hormones of the adrenal cortex are essential for life. They are divided into three different types as follows:

Mineralocorticoids. These hormones have to do with control of sodium, chloride, potassium, and other electrolytes. In a deficiency of the adrenal cortex (Addison's disease), there is a lack of aldosterone, one of the mineralocorticoids, which causes a reduction in sodium reabsorption from the kidneys. Subsequently, a reduction in the serum sodium, extracellular fluid volume, acidosis, potassium retention, and a fall in blood volume result in prompt development of a crisis.

Glucocorticoids. Cortisol, the principal secretion of the glucocorticoid zone of the cortex, helps in the maintenance of the normal blood sugar levels.

The mobilization of fats and proteins from tissues to form sugar is under the influence of cortisol as in melanin pigmentation of the skin. Proper amounts of cortisol for homeostasis (keeping an even keel) of the body are essential. Stress, whether produced by overeating, emotions, or illness, call for extra amounts of cortisol. Worry can cause all the symptoms of orally administered steroids (cortisone): muscle wasting, change in weight, nervous imbalance, poor healing, lymph node atrophy, poor clotting, etc.

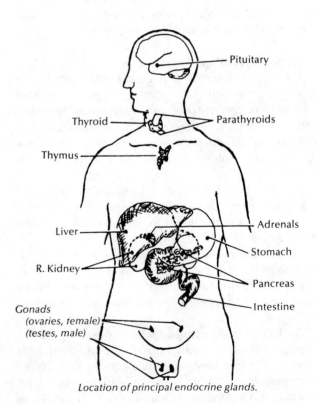

Location of principal endocrine glands.

Sex Hormones. Both androgens (male hormones) and estrogens (female hormones) are produced in the adrenal cortex. Both sexes produce both male and female hormones in the adrenal glands. The excess female hormones are detoxified in the liver of males, and the excess male hormones are detoxified in the liver of females. In liver disease, feminization of the male and masculinization of the female are possible.

Treatment with adrenal steroids increases hydrochloric acid secretion by the stomach. At the same time, excessive steroids interfere with the ability of the body to protect and heal itself and may result in serious peptic ulcer. Because the steroids mask symptoms of the ulcer, the lesion may progress to perforation or life-threatening hemorrhage before the victim is aware of what is happening. Treatment with adrenal steroids also reduces the ability of the body to produce an inflammatory reaction, thereby posing a hazard from all infectious organisms.

Thyroid

The thyroid is a small gland located in the neck just above the collar bone. It produces hormones, T-3 and T-4, that help regulate the rest of metabolism in every cell in the body.

Hyperthyroidism. Weight loss, an enlarged thyroid, bouts of diarrhea, a large appetite even in the presence of weight loss, mania, or other signs of nervousness or neurosis, increased body temperature, weakness, fine tremor of the tongue and fingers, increased blood pressure and pulse, and protruding eyes may all be signs of hyperthyroidism (too much thyroid hormone). Treatment for hyperthyroidism has three objectives: using up extra quantities of the hormone, depressing the activity of the gland, and treatment for possible inflammation of the gland.

1. Get plenty of outdoor exercise to use up excess thyroid hormone. Take the exercise in the cool of the day, being careful not to over exert. Judge the amount and intensity of the exercise by subjective signs.

2. Thiourea has the definite property of being able to reduce the function of the thyroid. It is known to be present in certain foods. The use of cabbage juice, since it is especially high in thiourea, may provide a convenient way to obtain a moderate quantity of the anti-thyroid component. Eat *at least* one serving daily of one or more of the following foods:

Cabbage	Rape seed
Carrots	Rutabaga
Kale	Soybean
Peaches	Spinach
Peanuts with skins on	Strawberries
Pears	Turnips

3. Avoid foods which contain pressor amines: sauerkraut (histamine), cheese (tyramine, tryptamine, and phenylethylamine), bananas (dopamine, norepinephrine, and serotonin), and wine (histamine and tyramine).

4. Avoid the use of iodized salt or other iodine.

5. Apply alternating hot and cold compresses to the thyroid area. This includes hot compresses molded to the neck and upper chest and maintained for six minutes. Alternate the hot with ice cold compresses for 30 seconds. Have three to five changes. Do this treatment twice daily for seven days, then only once a day in the morning for 30 days. In addition to helping normalize the function of the thyroid, this treatment will be helpful if there is inflammation in the gland causing it to be hyperactive.

6. Prolonged cold to the thyroid area, using an icebag for 30 minutes daily should be used in the mid-day, beginning from the first day of treatment with hot and cold compresses. The prolonged cold may suppress the activity of the thyroid.

7. If for some reason the alternating hot and cold compresses cannot be used, a heating compress or a charcoal poultice to the thyroid area each night may be substituted, or used in addition to that treatment.

8. For sedation, give a neutral bath for 40-90 minutes; the water should be neither hot nor cold (96-98 degrees).

9. Constipation and diarrhea may both be present, as the gastrointestinal tract tends to empty itself periodically and then be unresponsive. Use a cup of senna tea daily for constipation or better still, a small, cold enema. Use a three-ounce bulb syringe of cold tap water injected as an enema. Retain the water for one minute. This simple measure should initiate bowel movement. For diarrhea, use an ice bag to the abdomen or prolonged cold compresses. Take charcoal by mouth, about 4-8 tablets, twice daily. Charcoal tends to quiet the bowel and may adsorb some of the extra hormone.

Hypothyroidism. In prolonged or well-developed underfunction of the gland, the following symptoms are typical: constipation, an unusual sensitivity to chilling, a gain in weight, sallow complexion, a reddening of the hair in some cases, an elevation of cholesterol, anemia, a retention of fluids, hoarseness or deepening of the voice, and slow mental processes.

The treatment for an underfunctioning thyroid is as follows:

1. Use one serving of oats and bananas daily.

2. Avoid all foods containing thiourea (see list in the discussion of hyperthyroidism).

3. Use no free fats, sugars, or salts until the thyroid problem is under control. Blood fats tend to be abnormally elevated. Fluid tends to accumulate, especially if salt is used freely.

4. Use a 50-second cold shower to the adrenal areas morning and night followed by a "tapotement" (tapping with the fingertips by an attendant) over the area immediately beneath the shoulder blades to stimulate the adrenals. This will secondarily stimulate the thyroid. Use both hands for the tapotement, getting a hammermill action at the wrists and a regular rhythm between the two hands. Continue tapping about 30 seconds on each side.

5. Take a cool shower morning and evening as a cleansing bath and to stimulate metabolism.

6. Do not use an electric blanket, as the body metabolism will be slightly raised if the body must generate its own heat to keep warm in bed.

7. Get three to five hours of out-of-doors labor daily to stimulate the thyroid gland and elevate the metabolism.

8. Use a treatment of alternating hot and cold to the thyroid area as described under hyperthyroidism, mornings and evenings for seven days, then mornings only for 30 days. If this treatment cannot be done, a charcoal poultice to the thyroid area, worn for eight hours each night, can be substituted.

Some cases of hypothyroidism may involve virtual destruction of functional thyroid tissue by viral diseases, autoimmune processes, surgery, etc. In these cases, no improvement can be expected, and supplementation with natural or synthetic thyroid hormone substances is the only recourse. The supplements may, in fact, be lifesaving.

Cretinism. If an infant is born with a low thyroid function, the child may fail to clear physiologic jaundice within the usual five to ten days. He may fail to thrive, have mental and growth retardation, an enlarged tongue, a sallow complexion, coarse hair, and very slow reactions. The damage is irreversible; therefore, every effort should be made to diagnose and treat the disease in the first few weeks of life.

Menopause

There are several features of menopause that have a connection with diet. Vegetarian women are definitely at an advantage in handling menopause successfully.

Menopause occurs as early as age 35 and as late as age 60. There may be several years of irregular menstruation preceding the last period. Menopause cannot be said to have occurred until there has been no menstruation for twelve months or more. Post-menopausally, the reduction of estrogen that occurs from cessation of active ovarian function, results in the gradual shrinkage of the lining membranes of the vagina, the vulva, the uterus, and the fallopian tubes. A sensation of dryness, itching, and other symptoms may result. During the early years of menopause, eighty percent of women have hot flashes followed by cold sweats. The great majority of women, however, require no treatment whatever, as the symptoms are minor and will pass in a few weeks or months, or at the most, two or three years.

Contrary to popular misconceptions, menopause will not cause obesity, graying or thinning hair, wrinkled skin, cracking fingernails, varicose veins, flabby breast tissue, loss of muscle tone, tooth decay, hairiness, arthritis, high blood pressure, heart disease, or insomnia. These are all signs of aging, and in may instances can be slowed down by proper measures and sometimes reversed permanently. Neither frigidity nor unusual interest in sex is due to menopause, and will not be relieved by estrogen administration. Since the use of hormone preparations has been associated with serious health problems, it is recommended that the administration of hormones be avoided if at all possible. An increase in breast, ovarian, and endometrial cancer has been associated with the use of estrogens, both by injection and by mouth. Even vaginal creams and skin lotions and creams can greatly increase the blood levels of estrogens.

A group of foods has been found to be high in naturally occurring plant steroids similar in chemical formula to estrogen. As much as possible during the menopausal syndrome, some foods from each group should be used to fashion the menu for each meal. It has been demonstrated that when these foods are all withdrawn at once, a woman who is already post-menopausal may have withdrawal bleeding, illustrating that significant quantities of estrogenic compounds are present in the blood because of foods.

A woman who is going through menopause

may find these foods to be helpful in relieving symptoms. A man with prostate problems may find some relief from symptoms of enlargement or congestion by eating generously of these foods. For a list of foods high in plant steroids, see page 49. For fruit meals, select foods from the lists of fruits, grains, nuts, and seasonings. Other foods may be used to supplement these, and a search should be made for new listings of foods containing high plant steroid content.

The possibility of ingesting effective quantities of estrogen in the form of foods should be regarded more seriously. Beet roots, potato tubers, parsley roots, and yeast contain between 70 and 80 picograms of estrogen-like hormones per 100 grams (slightly less than ½ cup). Honey contains 40 to 600 International Units (I.U.) per kilogram. Dry sage contains 6,000 I.U. of estrogen per kilogram. Clover (*Trifolium subteranaeum*) fed to cattle as hay of fresh pasture contains estrogens in high enough concentrations to cause a slow delivery from uterine inertia in cattle, one of the functions of estrogen. Fasting removes estrogens that have been obtained from the foods and may cause amenorrhea in women. [231]

In addition to dietary control, we recommend that a woman obtain two to five hours of outdoor exercise daily in order to stimulate the ovaries and to achieve a sense of well-being. As an absolute minimum, twenty minutes daily of walking (if purposeful labor is not available) must be taken. The person should adjust the vigor of the exercise to her strength, but it should be described as "vigorous" for her.

An attempt should be made to avoid irritation of all mucous membranes, as these surfaces become quite thin following the menopause. When the vaginal opening is cleansed, the hands should be first washed and a lather left on the hands, which is used to thoroughly lather the area. Then plain, clear water, preferably a gentle spray, is used to meticulously rinse the area, being gentle and using no abrasive cloths. Blot dry. Generally one should not douche, as it can irritate, and regular douching for years has been associated with an increased incidence of cancer of the cervix.

A twenty minute, hot sitz bath daily, or hot compresses to the lower abdomen may be used to stimulate the ovaries. Continue this process for about thirty days.

Check clothing carefully for healthfulness. Girdles are taboo. There must be no band tight enough to leave a mark on the skin. Perhaps the most important item, yet the most difficult to attain, is warm clothing for the extremities. Even though there is no sensation of chilliness, the extremities should be warmly clothed. Blood loses much latent heat from a bare skin area. Experimentally, there is alteration of the blood flow in the pelvic organs if only one hand is chilled for five minutes.

Osteoporosis

Osteoporosis is a thinning of the bones, usually in the elderly or in invalids, leading to easy fracturing. Osteoporosis is very unlikely to occur in a vegetarian woman who gets plenty of exercise. Animal products cause the blood to become slightly acid, and acids are well-known to dissolve or etch metals. Calcium is no exception, and the slightest acid condition of the blood produced by the acid wastes from animal products dissolves calcium from the bones, causing osteoporosis.

The pull of muscles on bones and the jolting of the bones resulting from walking or running, stimulates the bones to attract and hold more calcium. The essentiality of exercise to prevent calcium loss was brought vividly to our attention by the experiences of the first astronauts. In the few hours they spent circling the earth in a weightless condition, there was a significant loss of bone calcium; the markedly increased loss of calcium in the urine raised fears of possible kidney stones. An elaborate system of exercises was devised for later space flights, and the problem has been lessened. Exercise is even more important in the elderly than in the youthful person in order to keep the bones in good condition.

Causes of Osteoporosis

Alcohol   Steroids (synthetic)

Causes of Osteoporosis, continued

High uric acid in blood
Pancreatic disease
Liver disease
High blood fats
Birth control pills
Gaucher's Disease
Caisson's Disease
fractures and dislocations of bones
Smoking
Coffee *(1 cup per day causes 1.4% skeletal calcium loss per year after the age of 50)*

Synthetic thyroid supplements in excess; *or--*
Overactive thyroid
Subtotal Gastrectomy
Excessive intake of vitamins A or D
Excessive intake of salt, phosphorus, protein, or sugar
Antacids containing aluminum
Long term use of tetracycline type antibiotics

High Phosphorus Sources

Processed meats
Red meats
Potatoes
Brewers yeast
Detergents on unrinsed dishes

Instant soups
Soft drinks
Processed cheese
Baking powder products

CHAPTER FIFTEEN

Diabetes, the Principle Disease of Metabolism

Accelerated Aging

Diabetes is a true degenerative disease; it might be designated as a "nutritional degenerative disease." Diabetes can very properly be considered to accelerate aging. The scope of the problem involved in diabetes is enormous. Today it is generally estimated by the most conservative people that there are at least five million people in the United States who are diagnosed as having diabetes. A recent interview with Dr. George Cahill, president of the American Diabetes Association, gave this figure as the current estimate. Certainly, the number of diabetics that are as yet undiagnosed would be at least twice as many and perhaps three times as many as the already recognized diabetics. Everyone agrees that the disease is increasing rapidly. Diabetes has been the subject of intense interest, research, and screening for many years; physicians and laity alike have been aware of the increase over the last several decades.

Diabetes represents two separate diseases. They behave differently, as a doctor sees them, although they have certain similar characteristics. The two types of diabetes are "juvenile diabetes" and "maturity onset diabetes." Juvenile refers to childhood onset diabetes, more commonly referred to now as "insulin-dependent", or Type 1, diabetes, since it can begin in the adult also. Maturity onset diabetes is referred to as "non-insulin dependent," or Type II. Of the two, the juvenile onset is more serious. In years past, it has ended fatally in most cases, sometimes in just a few months. The person has an absolute lack of insulin. If diabetes is untreated, the health declines rapidly and the patient dies. Before the discovery of insulin in the early 1920's, there was no satisfactory treatment for this type of diabetes, which meant that these children

soon died. They first lost weight rapidly in spite of eating voraciously; then they sank into a coma and died. At autopsy, they sometimes showed advanced atrophy of the beta cells of the pancreas.

The pancreas is the organ primarily involved, but only the *endocrine* function of the pancreas is affected in this disease. It is quite interesting that before 1920 we had only a faint notion that the pancreas was involved in diabetes or that the pancreas even had a hormonal or endocrine function. There is also an *exocrine* function that produces the digestive enzymes lipase, amylase, and trypsin, which are secreted into the pancreatic duct and delivered to the small intestine. In the endocrine function, the secretions go directly into the blood stream. They are transported directly across the membrane of the cell into the capillaries without passing through a duct or tube. When Doctors Best and Banting were attempting to find the agent that would lower blood sugar, they had a struggle to isolate insulin even in its crude form. It was quite a dramatic event.

Insulin replacement, strictly speaking, is not a drug medication, although it is foreign to the body using it because the type we now use is made by an animal. In recent years, scientists have been able to work out the structural formula for human insulin and to synthesize it. Pure human insulin should be a vast improvement. In the past, some diabetics have become allergic to the various types of animal insulin. As yet, we know of no allergies to human insulin. With tremendously improved techniques made possible by genetic engineering, supplies should become much more plentiful and inexpensive in the near future.

In the past, several oral antidiabetic agents have been tried. Most doctors have become disenchanted with them as they are not very effective, and they appear to accelerate the complications of diabetes, especially in the cardiovascular field. They are not effective in juvenile onset diabetes. Dr. Jack Davidson, of Emory University School of Medicine, and other authorities believe they are actually *contraindicated*. Dr. Davidson says that 90-100% of overweight adult-onset diabetics can and should be controlled by diet alone. Anemia has been reported in patients taking oral anti-diabetic agents, because of supression of the bone marrow. The names of the agents are Diabenese, Orinase, Dymelor, and Tolinase.[232] Diabenese has also been reported to cause severe low blood sugar, to the point of coma, as well as liver damage and jaundice.[233]

There is an hereditary component to diabetes. However, in recent years there have been some interesting findings to suggest that much of this disorder is acquired rather than inherited. Perhaps in many people there is a latent tendency to diabetes that is inherited, but as long as a person maintains a good diet, that tendency will not be manifested. However, if he indulges in an improper diet, such as the average American diet, he is likely to develop diabetes as time goes on. An interesting work that Dr. Cahill refers to in the interview cited is the possibility of viral diseases triggering diabetes. There is an abundance of evidence to support this thesis. What seems to happen is that the virus or viruses, perhaps a number of them, enter the beta cells of the pancreas which produce insulin. It may be that they actually infect them and destroy the beta cells, or perhaps injure them is such a way as to produce an autoimmune disease. That is, they cause a sort of allergic reaction against the body's own tissues which causes the destruction or impairment of function of the beta cells.

Some studies have been published recently concerning identical twins, one of whom has developed juvenile onset diabetes and the other has not. Identical twins are identical in heredity. If one twin develops an hereditary disease, it is expected that the other will develop the same disease. There have been, however, quite a few cases described in which one twin develops diabetes and the other twin does not. This suggests that perhaps a virus may be followed a few months later with an outbreak of juvenile diabetes. Influenza, pneumonia, scarlet fever, and other diseases have also been implicated.

The Pima Indians

It has been observed that the stress of illness, accident, or personal tragedy may precipitate diabetes that has been smoldering for years. One in 2500 individuals under the age of fifteen has diabetes. It is estimated that 10-30 million adults have diabetes, either preclinical or clinical. It is impressive that 80% of overweight adults eventually develop diabetes. In recent decades there has occurred what is called a "diabetes explosion." What has caused the vast increase in diabetes, especially the adult onset type seen in the Western world today? This question has been the stimulus for many epidemiological studies in recent years, of which we cite only three which most clearly point up the cause:

First, the Pima Indians in their ordinary enviroment had no known diabetes. Since they have come onto reservations and are eating a diet high in sugar and refined carbohydrates, 40-50% of the tribe have overt diabetes. This is due both to the change in their diet and also to the fact that they exercise much less and are much fatter now than they have been in the past several decades.

The Yemenite Jews

The next study has been described a number of times. An Israeli physician, in a speech before the American Chemical Society, incriminated sugar as one of the greatest problems of our civilization today. In fact, he said governments should put a danger warning on sugar packages just as on cigarettes! He gave the example of the Yemenite Jews, among whom diabetes was virtually unknown two or three decades ago. However at present, one out of five adult Yemeni living in Israel over the age 30 have diabetes! The principle change in their lifestyle has been a marked increase in sweets and sugar.

The Eskimos and Diabetes

The third study is probably the most graphic, involving the Eskimo. The entire issue of *Nutrition Today* for November-December, 1971, was devoted to nutrition in Canada with a large portion of it describing the Eskimos. The article was written by a physician who had lived with and studied these people for two or three decades. A graph showed the average intake of sugar in all forms, by pounds, in 1959 to 1967. In 1959, the average intake per year, per person, among the Eskimos in Canada was 26 pounds. Just eight years later, in 1967, it was 104.2 pounds! The percentage of their total carbohydrate intake from cereals and flour-- that is, the unrefined carbohydrates--dropped for 82% to 55%. Eskimos have been noted through the years for their strong and beautiful teeth. Older women's teeth were worn off almost to the gum line because of chewing hides for making of leather. These stubs of teeth used to be free of caries and in very good condition. Now, in contrast, those who live close to the trading posts have teeth which are entirely decayed; only blackened snags remain. Instead of chewing caribou hides, they chew on caramels and chocolates and drink soda pop, beginning in infancy with a nipple on a soda pop bottle. When children's teeth erupt, they have already developed caries.

In addition to dental disease, other problems are appearing. One is growth acceleration. Eskimos are getting much taller. It used to be said that growth acceleration in children in developing countries was due to increased consumption of protein. It is known that this is not the case with Eskimos, whose protein consumption has actually gone down markedly as their refined carbohydrates have gone up; it appears that sugar has upset the metabolic system of youngsters. The children are getting taller and heavier due to stimulation of the entire glandular system, including growth hormones. Eskimo children are going through puberty two or three years earlier than before 1950. Many nutritionists believe that this is one of the major factors contributing to the social, mental, and emotional problems young people have today. While the children are physically mature, the social and emotional make up is not at all mature.

Prior to a few years ago, diabetes was virtually unknown among Eskimos. More new cases of diabetes have been discovered in one group of Eskimos living in the Canadian western Arctic during one three year period than occurred in Eskimos in all of Canada a few years ago. There is also marked increase in gallbladder disease. Prior to the 1950's, one main hospital in Canada received all Eskimos who were referred for various operations. No cholecystectomies had ever been reported in an Eskimo before 1950. Now, operations for gallbladder disease outnumber *all other operations*. Acne, which was formerly unknown in Eskimos, has greatly increased. Now it has become quite common, just as in the United States.

The current intake of sugar in the United States has been estimated at 120 to 140 pounds per person, per year, equivalent to about 35-40 teaspoons a

day. This change in diet has come about over some 80-100 years, but the comparable change in the Eskimos occurred in less than a decade.

The classic symptoms of full-blown diabetes are "polydipsia, polyuria, and polyphagia" (much drinking, much urination, and much eating). Yet despite much eating, the individual may lose weight and strength. Often there are itching of the skin, vaginal infections, urinary tract infections, other infections, slow wound healing, changes in vision, wide mood swings, and many other symptoms.

The complications of diabetes represent one of the major problems that physicians face. An increase occurs in all types of blood vessel problems in the eye, the legs, the brain, the kidneys, and the heart of those with diabetes. Coronary heart attacks are much more common among diabetics. The juvenile diabetic generally dies about 30 years early unless given special care. The better the control of the blood sugar in the diabetic, the fewer the complications, and the longer the life.

Glucose is normally handled by the body in four different ways: It may be utilized for work energy immediately, converted to glycogen for liver storage, converted to fat, or converted to muscle glycogen. During a glucose tolerance test, a diabetic shows a rapid rise in blood sugar to a very high level and a slow return to normal, meaning that glucose was not handled well in these four pathways. Within two hours, a non-diabetic will have been able to return his blood sugar to the normal level. The diabetic shows a delay, perhaps an hour or more, in returning to the fasting level. Generally, as the non-diabetic's blood sugar falls, it will slightly overshoot the fasting level and go below that level for a short while. The return of the blood sugar to normal is a function of the combined influences of insulin, glucagon (which keeps the blood sugar level from going too low), the action of the stomach emptying, the rate at which digestion occurs in the first ten inches of the small bowel, and the action of the liver. (*See chapter on digestion.*) Insulin promotes the uptake of glucose from the intestine and its utilization by the cells for energy or other uses. Insulin also promotes the transport of amino acids through the cell membrane in much the same carrier system that glucose is transported.

Formerly it was taught that a diabetic must markedly restrict his carbohydrate, starches, and sugars. The older dieticians concentrated on fats and proteins, while restricting carbohydrates. Dieticians now agree that this approach is wrong. A diabetic can get along quite well on as much as 60-

80% of his total calories as carbohydrates (starchy foods), provided they are in the unrefined forms of cereals, fruits, grains, and nuts. In these foods, carbohydrates are slowly absorbed. They do not raise the blood sugar abruptly as do refined starches and sugars.

Reduction in weight is of primary importance in treating maturity onset diabetes. The proper number of calories for weight loss will vary with the person. Perhaps 1000, 1200, or 1500 calories will be required, determined by the age, weight, sex, and the amount of energy expended each day. If the weight can be reduced to somewhat below the normal for the patient's age and sex, he will usually respond better. We find that patients live longer and have fewer complications on this diet than on the higher fat and protein diets. Also they are more comfortable as the larger quantities of food produce a greater sense of satisfaction with meals.

Dr. Davidson, working in the diabetic clinic of Grady Hospital in Atlanta, has devised an interesting approach to treatment of the poorly controlled, obese, adult-onset diabetic. Research has shown that many of these patients produce sufficient insulin, but that it is not utilized properly. Apparently, the insulin receptors in the membranes of the cells become insensitive and cannot bind insulin so that it can be used in overweight persons. Dr. Davidson found a number in this category who were taking over 100 units of insulin daily, yet were poorly controlled, with blood sugars regularly running in the range of 300-500 mg percent (ideal for normal people should average 70-85). He brought a group of them into the hospital, stopped their insulin abruptly, and put them on a total fast for up to five days. Blood sugars were checked regularly. In nearly all, the blood sugar fell into the normal range within three to five days with no ill effects. They were then restarted on a very restricted diet, averaging 800-1000 calories a day. In several cases, the blood sugar remained normal, and in every case the level was much better than it had been before the fast even while still on the huge doses of insulin! Apparently the cellular receptors had been "reset" by the fast. We have tried this approach in a number of cases and have been quite pleased with the results. We do not recommend that this be tried in an unsupervised enviroment however, as an occasional diabetic will experience a rise in blood sugar and will go into acidosis and possibly could go into coma, if insulin is not promptly restarted.

Since adult onset diabetes is characterized by being overweight, the only treatment needed in most instances is that of sustained weight loss to a normal weight, or preferably, about 10% below the normal weight ("ideal weight"). Insulin is rarely if ever required. The diet should be strict, sufficient to maintain nutritional balance, but appropriate for proper weight loss. A period of fasting may be desirable, particularly in the early phases, to assist the individual in appetite control. The juvenile diabetic, however, may accumulate ketone bodies in the blood during a fast, develop acidosis, and quickly enter a crisis. For this reason, juvenile diabetics should not be fasted, except with skilled supervision.

Juvenile Diabetes

Insulin is essential for the transfer of glucose into the cycle that creates energy. Insulin is the facilitator to get sugar into the cell. If insulin is not there, the person starves to death, even though he has plenty of food. Although juvenile diabetes can occur at any age, the typical time of onset is at the time a young person begins to be subject to the many stresses associated with adolescence, or around the age of twelve. Dr. Cahill spoke of having seen a Spanish-American War veteran, nearly 100 years old, with what was described as typical juvenile onset diabetes. On the other hand, he said that we are now seeing typical *maturity onset* diabetes in six-, seven-, and eight-year-old fat children, illustrating that there is an overlap in age. Nevertheless, under the age of twenty, the likelihood is overwhelming that beginning diabetes is of the juvenile onset variety. The incidence of these diseases is important because only about 10% of diabetics are of the childhood type, which means more than 90% of cases are of the adult onset type. This makes the childhood type diabetes relatively rare. An occasional person recovers from juvenile diabetes, usually early in its course. The reason recovery occurs in some is not known, but we believe immediate treatment with well-regulated rest, exercise, study periods, and the application of hydrotherapy and other simple remedies, begun as soon as the diagnosis is made, with a carefully controlled simple vegetarian diet increases the opportunity that the acute disease will not become chronic diabetes.

It is rare that a juvenile diabetic can be taken entirely off insulin. Nevertheless, in many cases, a very small dosage of insulin can be used, and with a strict diet, the individual can be maintained in good control, helping prevent or delay the onset of serious degenerative disease.

The juvenile diabetic has a greater likelihood of

developing both insulin reactions and diabetic acidosis, due to poor control of the blood sugar level and resulting faulty metabolic processes.

The diabetic should especially guard his health to avoid infections of any kind: respiratory, gastro-intestinal, dermal (particularly of the feet), and genitourinary. The feet should be given special attention and regular pedicures. A very small injury or lesion on the foot becomes a major problem for the diabetic, whereas, for the non-diabetic it may represent an insignificant matter. Since protein breakdown is increased over that of a normal person, and protein synthesis is decreased, wound healing may be delayed in some diabetics.

The Hypoglycemic Syndrome Defined

The most common disorder in the United States today is that of "accelerated aging," also called the "hypoglycemic syndrome." Hans Selye, the world's best known authority on stress, has called the same disorder the "general adaptation syndrome." This syndrome is a degenerative disease state. It evolves in this way: A mother who often has a history of diabetes in her family, gains perhaps 40, 50 or 60 pounds during a pregnancy, gives birth to a baby weighing eight pounds or more (a sign of diabetes, and the heavier the baby, the greater the risk). The disorder often begins in the hospital nursery with the feeding of sugar water between formula feedings. When the child is brought home from the hospital, he is often on as rich a formula as can be tolerated. Shortly the baby begins taking large amounts of rich food. From the beginning the problem forces maximal growth, the earliest possible sexual development, and the earliest possible psychological and mental maturation. The child is able to comprehend reading early and starts to school before development is sufficiently advanced to withstand the stresses of school. Throughout childhood, there is too little exercise, too much sugar, too many concentrated foods, too much protein, and usually too much salt. The child grows up rapidly, sometimes experiencing fatigue alternating with hyperactivity, which is considered to be normal. There may be excessive dental caries. He may have a bout of appendicitis before the age of twelve. He has constipation from time to time. Then, as he grows older, he does well in school, matures more rapidly than the boys of his father's and grandfather's generation, and girls begin their menstrual periods at an average age of 11.7 years (the average was 16.2 years in 1880). With the onset of early maturation often comes a serious problem

with appetite and weight control. It has been postulated that breast feeding teaches appetite control better than formula feeding, as the child becomes accustomed to having the less rich foods with the first part of the meal and the richest foods for the finish. Salads and less concentrated foods could be taken first, with a small quantity of richer food (even breads are sufficient) at the end of the meal, for best appetite control. A lifelong battle begins with weight gain in infancy, due to the artificial formula, and becomes acute during adolescence.

Often the child becomes a good student, but develops in the early teens the unrest and wanderlust so characteristic of prematurely sexually developed American children. Because of early maturation, the child may become a dropout from school as he feels himself ready to select a job and become independent of the counsel of his parents. Often he may experience the "nesting instinct" with its desire to choose a mate and settle down for life. The early flash of brilliance seen in the precocious childhood dwindles with a splash of unwise choices and poor judgment in the mid and late teenage years.

Normally, less than two teaspoons of "sugar" (glucose) circulate in the blood at any one time. A small amount of sugar is stored, however, in the liver, muscles, skin, and kidneys but very little in the brain. The brain needs to have a steady, second-by-second supply, or mental problems such as nervousness, anxiety, irritability, depression, forgetfulness, confusion, indecisiveness, poor concentration, nightmares, and suicidal tendencies result. Many of these patients naturally are referred to the psychiatrist, but thousands of others struggle along with their symptoms. When the blood sugar drops, the brain sends an SOS to the adrenals whose hormone releases glucose from the liver and muscles. Eventually the adrenals begin to be depleted. Caffeine, nicotine, and alcohol also stimulate the adrenals, and in those who use these substances, the symptoms are enhanced (most distressingly the mental symptoms) and the aging process accelerated.

Therefore, in the midteen years, the person may experience, for the first time, a blue or depressed period. Since it is usually merely an overreaction to a real, and not an imagined situation, nobody gets concerned. These small depressions may be simple affairs, not causing much trouble other than an intensification of what is considered standard operating procedure in a modern household--teenage rebellion. An early marriage is often contracted, and the stage is set for a lifetime during which the shadows never lift from their unhappy home. Children begin to be born into the home. If the symptomatic individual is a woman, which is more than a 50% likelihood, she experiences an increase in "all gone" feelings, headaches, fast heart beat, fatigue, allergies, digestive tract symptoms, hemorrhoids, mental confusion, and inability to organize her work. If there is no change in lifestyle, the condition may eventually progress to bizzare thoughts and compulsions with intolerable physical symptoms such as shooting pains, skin burns, and scalp symptoms including such sensations as water dripping on the scalp, pressure inside the head, or a band around the scalp. There are always gastro-intestinal symptoms if they are searched for, although many patients overlook these since they have been present since the dawn of memory. Although she is intelligent, she begins to lose her various interests in life. In fact, she may have partly withdrawn from society because she does not feel well enough to enjoy other people's company. She is often in bed, and she never has energy to do anything with the children or with her husband; she becomes somewhat of a non-entity. Her husband recognizes that he must take over certain duties, such as the rearing of the children, and taking care of certain social obligations. Mother sort of retires and is no longer really effective as either wife or mother. If she does maintain her duties, she is often hard to please, moody, irritable, and frequently exasperated.

She visits a doctor who checks her out physically and finds no organic illness. As he is trained to accept indications of frank disease only, he does not usually recognize the small indications from the laboratory tests that the biochemistries are trending in a wrong direction. When we examine laboratory reports, we recognize three categories of results: abnormal, average, and ideal. We find these individuals to be more likely to be outside of the ideal range for several of their biochemistries as follows: cholesterol levels above 100 plus the age; triglycerides above 100; uric acid above 5 mg for a woman and 6 mg for a man; hemoglobin readings at sea level between 10.5 and 12.5 gm for a woman, 12.5 and 14.5 for men; and fasting blood sugar levels of 70-85. If a glucose tolerance test is done, at 30 minutes the person may have 120; in one hour 165; at two hours 102; at three hours perhaps 80; at four hours 47; and at five hours 68. This would be one type of typical blood sugar pattern. At the two hour level, there may be a trace of sugar in the urine. Two of the blood sugar levels were low. Many physicians still may say that there is no metabolic problem

demonstrated, if that level is not lower than about 58%. The patient may be sent home with the instruction that the only thing wrong is "in your head." Just get out more, spend more time with other people, and take up your duties as you should. Everything will be all right. The husband of our patient is informed of the impressions that nothing serious is wrong, and that she must try harder to feel well.

After another year or so and another baby or two, she begins to have really bizarre thoughts. One of our patients wondered what might happen if she were to put her child in the washing machine. She knew she would never do such a thing, but the thought became an obsession that occupied her mind. Another of our patients described her thoughts when she went to the bank. Her only thought was an obsession: "What if I had come here to rob this bank?" She would become hysterical and could not stay even to do her banking, but would literally run from the bank in great distress. She finally came to the point that she could not even drive her automobile.

The obsessions come because of a lack of mental energy to change the thoughts and to concentrate on proper mental activity. There is an imbalance of inhibitory and facilitative nerve cell influences in the brain. She expresses some of her compulsive thoughts to her husband which may shake his confidence in her. He takes her to another physician and hears the suggestion that she should visit the psychiatrist. She rejects the idea initially, because she recognizes that she is quite capable of discernment and doing normal perspective and judgmental activities. Nevertheless, there *are* the obsessive thoughts and the inability to get organized. At last she accepts the idea that she has a psychiatric illness and goes hopefully for treatment. She may be given electroshock therapy or heavy tranquilizing medication.

Even though she may sense some improvement for a while, due to a placebo effect and a great desire and need to be well and perform her duties, eventually she has a return of the same symptoms, but now more disheartening. She may have been gradually gaining weight. She has periodic cravings for sweets which have been present for years. She gets weakness and trembling before meals. She is thoroughly miserable. Eventually she reads a book or magazine article on the subject of "hypoglycemia," recognizes herself in this description, manages to get the diagnostic laboratory tests, and the diagnosis is confirmed.

Not every case is exactly as we have presented

here. There are fairly wide variations on this basic theme. A professional man may tell you he no longer has any ambition to continue his work. A mother may walk out and leave three little children and a husband, to take a job and a small apartment in a distant city. Many a person has come to my office saying: "I am at the end of my rope. I have been to fifteen doctors before you. If you do not have some help for me, I think I will walk into the Chattahoochee River until it just covers me over." It is quite a satisfaction to see such individuals receive help and begin to be relieved of unhappy symptoms which have been regular companions for years.

Treatment for Diabetes and the Hypoglycemic Syndrome

The treatment for juvenile and adult onset diabetes, as well as the hypoglycemic syndrome, is very similar. A two-meal plan is ideal, and the upper limit of eating experiences one may have in one day is three. The five to seven meals daily often prescribed for this condition merely prolong the affliction and urge along the onset of degenerative disease. A substantial breakfast and lunch should be taken. Supper, if eaten, should be only whole grains or fruit. There should be at least five hours between meals. The mealtime should not be varied by so much as a few minutes. The time one eats is fully as important as what is eaten.

Many advise high protein feedings between meals, with bedtime snacks and even eating during the night. This practice is unphysiological and invariably promotes digestive upsets. The pancreas and stomach have been over-stimulated for years and they need rest. They should have to work only at specified intervals, so that they can recover their rythmical pattern. Therefore, mealtimes should be very regular, with as little variation as possible, and nothing eaten between meals. Individuals who have reactive hypoglycemia (over 90%) have absolutely no problem in maintaining adequate blood sugar levels between meals or while fasting. Their problem comes two to four hours after eating sweets or highly refined, rapidly absorbed carbohydrates. Avoidance of these items, and any article of diet to which one may be sensitive or allergic, with the substitution of a proper diet and health program, solves the "ping-pong" swings in blood sugar. When the blood sugar goes high, the pancreas senses the situation and throws out a large load of insulin, which overcorrects the high blood sugar level, and the blood sugar falls too low. Many symptoms may

occur at that time, but most come later as a result of altered metabolism. One should recognize that the over-reactive pancreas cannot immediately correct itself, and some symptoms may persist for weeks or months, even on an excellent program. We have seen an occasional patient who was unable to tolerate even the bland or tart fruits for several months, but had to consume a vegetable-whole grain diet for a while.

We do not promote the high protein meat substitutes for patients with this syndrome; these foods are usually too concentrated for them. We recommend that if they use them, it should be in stews or roasts so that a small quantity of the meat substitute is distributed in a large pot of food. The more highly concentrated the food, the more difficulty these individuals will have. Of course, animal products, especially cheese, are also highly concentrated, and prolong the difficulties experienced.

The hypothalamus may control appetite by storing glucose. In hypoglycemia, the hypothalamus cannot store glucose, and the person cannot control his appetite. Sucrose increases the liver synthesis of cholesterol.

For our patients with the hypoglycemic syndrome or diabetes, we allow whole grain breads. They are easily handled by the digestive apparatus. Our patients do well with whole grain breads, despite the aversion with which they are often regarded. It is white breads, white rice, and other refined grains that cause a problem, but the whole grain products should not be restricted. We advise that all animal products be left out of the diet, at least in the beginning, and whole grains take the place of these items to good advantage. Whole grain cooked cereals are excellent, but no boxed or refined cereals are allowed, not even cream of wheat, which has part of the bran removed. Vegetables may be used in liberal quantities.

We advise that no dairy products be used. Milk is high in lactose, (milk sugar), and is constipating; many individuals who have this syndrome already have constipation. Gastrointestinal problems are so frequently seen with the hypoglycemic syndrome that we believe that they aften precede the metabolic problems as the very first part of the syndrome. Unsweetened milk substitutes (nut and soy milk) may be used. *Eat for Strength* cookbook has many suitable recipes for persons with accelerated aging syndrome. The commercial soy milks should not be used because of their high sugar content. One glass of commercial soy milk contains almost three teaspoons of sugar.

Green and black ripe olives and avocados may be used. Nuts and seeds may be used sparingly, but should not be used in large quantities because of their concentrated nature. We allow coffee and tea substitutes; the herb teas are quite acceptable. We believe that people will be happier on the diet if they make the decision not to become dependent on artificial sweeteners. We instruct patients to learn to make their own salad dressings, savory foods, and fruit dishes, and not to depend for enjoyment of food on such things as highly sweetened desserts. The person should not allow what he *cannot* eat to spoil his relish for what he *can* eat. For every item he must give up, there are a hundred foods he will find delightful if effort is put forth toward finding them. The patient should bear in mind that millions of people the world over eat regularly a simple diet with great relish, and this experience will soon be his if a little persistence to reeducate the appetite is practiced.

Caffeine and nicotine are potent stimulators of insulin production and must be absolutely avoided. The same thing is true of alcohol, which is a concentrated carbohydrate, a pancreatic stimulator, as well as a specific protoplasmic poison for all cells, especially the pancreatic cells. Drink plenty of water between meals—enough to keep the urine almost colorless. For most people, this will average six to eight glasses a day. Drink water no closer than about 15 minutes before meals, and wait about 30 minutes after meals. Generally the less fluids taken with meals the better. Follow the suggestion for a proper diet for the accelerated aging syndrome, diabetes and "hypoglycemia."

Diets high in pectin from fruits reduce the level of blood sugar after a meal.[234] Diets low in fats cause a lowering of the blood sugar in diabetes and a reduction of sugar in the urine, often eliminating all urine sugar excretion.[235] When a simple diet of fruits, vegetables, and whole grains is given in a way to induce weight loss, and coupled with exercise and regularity, most diabetics over forty will be rewarded by complete control of the diabetes without insulin. The program should be carefully followed as the stakes are high.

Foods Allowed

Breads. Whole grain breads, plain corn bread, or hoecake. Use only unleavened or yeast breads; baking powder and soda have an irritating effect, both on the gastrointestinal tract and other organ systems. Make your own whole wheat melba toast by drying slices of whole wheat bread in the oven (see *Eat For Strength* cookbook for recipes) and whole grain crackers.

Cooked Cereals. Oatmeal, steel-cut oats, granola made without honey, wheat cereals, buckwheat, barley, millet, brown rice, grits, soy spaghetti, and whole wheat macaroni.

Vegetables. All may be used in liberal quantities, except those with a high sugar content listed under foods to avoid.

Milk Substitutes. Nut milks, soy milk made from soy flour or soy beans (not commercial soy milks which are sweetened), cheeses made from nuts, flours, or vegetables; sour and sweet creams made from healthful recipes.

Miscellaneous. Green and black olives (not stuffed), avocado.

Nuts and Seeds. All kinds may be used, as well as their butters (peanut butter, almond butter, and sesame butter), but should be used sparingly. Use raw or lightly roasted nuts and seeds.

Coffee and Tea Substitutes. Postum, Caphag, Pero, Breakfast Cup, etc. All herb teas are also acceptable.

Artificial Sweeteners. Use in small amounts, not more than the equivalent of three teaspoons of sugar daily. It is best to learn to eat foods in their natural, unsweetened state as much as possible.

Fruits. All fresh fruits except the very sweet ones; all canned fruits in water pack or natural juices. There is some evidence that in some people fruits do not raise the blood sugar as high as comparable quantities of vegetables.[236] Some are fearful of using fruits, but unless they have been concentrated by drying or by adding sugar, there is usually no problem. The availability of carbohydrates from vegetables is generally as great or greater than from fruits, although it would seem that fruits with their high sugar content would give more sugars to the blood than a vegetable meal. One study showed grain to yield the largest amount of carbohydrate for blood sugar, vegetables next, and fruits lowest.[237,238]

Foods to Avoid

Sugars. White, brown, or raw sugar, honey, syrups, jams, jellies, preserves, jello, etc.

Pastries. Pies, cakes, any sweetened desserts.

Refined Grains. White bread, buns, white melba toast, crackers, and saltines, cakes, cookies, macaroni, spaghetti, white rice, boiled corn meal, etc.

Sweetened Fruits and Vegetables. Eat sparingly of all dried fruit, especially raisins, dates, and figs. Bananas, mangoes, watermelon, and sweet potatoes must be eaten sparingly. Some do better to avoid these very sweet foods altogether.

Caffeine Drinks. Coffee, teas, colas, and chocolate, even Sanka and Decaf. Very small quantities of caffeine improperly stimulate the pancreas.

Soft Drinks. All kinds, including Kool-aid, bottled drinks, fruit juices.

Dry Cereals. Granola made with honey; all boxed cereals.

Tobacco. In all forms.

Condiments. Spices, vinegar, pickles, relish, mustard, catsup, hot pepper, commercial mayonnaise.

Cheeses. Except those noted under *Foods Allowed.*

Medicines containing Caffeine. Among the common ones are: Anacin, APC, BC, Cafergot, Cope, Coricidin, Dolar, Empirin Compound, Excedrin, Fiorinal, Four Way Cold Tablets, Stanback, Trigesic, and Vanquish. Nicotine is related to caffeine and often has a profound effect on the pancreas.

Exercise is the best friend of one with accelerated aging syndrome. It helps keep the appetite under control, it neutralizes stress, lowers blood cholesterol, promotes digestion and normalizes blood sugar. Make it your daily companion. Breathe deeply, and meditate on nature as you walk.

Ellen White published the symptoms of hypoglycemia many years before it was recognized as a clinical syndrome: faintness, nasal catarrh (hay fever), fatigue, headaches, bad taste in the mouth, etc. She also recommended the two-meal plan as a specific remedy, along with the simple dietary and the prescription for regularity and outdoor labor.

Questions Often Asked About the Hypoglycemic Syndrome

Question: Is there a way to have palatable soy milk without buying the commercial product?

Answer: Eat For Strength has substitute recipes for various milks, creams, cheeses, cottage cheese, other dairy products, and scrambled eggs using soybeans, nuts, and cereal grains.

Question: What is wrong if soy milk causes gas?

Answer: It may be that too great a quantity is taken. If any food causes gas there are several things to do. First, reduce the quantity of food to a very small amount to see if that amount can be tolerated. Second, chew to a cream any gas-forming food before swallowing it. In case of liquids, hold a small sip in the mouth until well mixed with saliva. Third, take no beverages, liquid food, or water with the meal. Depend on saliva to keep the food

generously moistened. Drinking plenty of water between meals will ensure adequate saliva for meals. Taking small bites will enable the chewing to do its proper work of moistening and grinding. At first, great effort and attention will be needed to break the habit of large bites and swallowing before the food has become thoroughly ground. This is the hardest single habit to break when adopting a new lifestyle.

Question: Is the small amount of sugar in soyonnaise made from Soyagen all right for a diabetic to use?

Answer: Yes, in most cases, since in the making of the soyannaise from Soyagen, a half cup of the powder is used to two cups of water. Less than two cups of oil and some lemon juice will go in also. Of that, your serving is at most a tablespoon. That is not a significant quantity of sugar, except for a person with severe hypoglycemia. I have a greater objection to the oil, which, for most diabetics is more injurious than the sugar. It should be constantly remembered that the problem is with all concentrated nutrients, not just sugars; and that fats are handled in the body in a very special way because of their potential for causing damage or reducing tissue oxygenation. A trial with an oil free diet will convince most people of the physiologic advantages of eating no free fats.

Question: How long is the diet to be continued?

Answer: We recommend that no deviation be allowed for the first twelve months. Most people will require a year or more to recover. Many will receive benefit after a few days on the program. Others will not begin to see any improvement until they have been on the program for several months. Even after one is "cured," there remains forever a weakness, and a return to the old habits will often bring a return of symptoms or an advance in deterioration with a vengence. After twelve full months, gradually add some of the sweet fruits. If symptoms such as a headache or weakness and trembling before the next meal return it would be obvious that recovery is not yet fully achieved. Every person is an individual, and some trial and error is to be expected.

There are some people who can use some dried fruit, such as apricots or peaches. Eliminate everything questionable at first, and then, very cautiously, put back one thing at a time.

Soft drinks should all be left off. Fruit juices have quite a lot of natural sugar. An eight-ounce glass may contain two or three teaspoons of sugar, both fructose and sucrose, as well as other sugars, making a considerable quantity of easily absorbed carbohydrate.

Question: Why is caffeine not good for diabetics or hypoglycemics?

Answer: Caffeine is far more damaging to the human body than we have before recognized. Caffeine, particularly, injures the islets of Langerhans in the pancreas where insulin is produced. Even Sanka and Decaf should be avoided, although they have only about 15-18 mg of caffeine per cup.

Caffeine

Adenine

Caffeine and adenine (a non-poisonous purine base, a chemical component of every cell nucleus) are very close together in molecular structure. Because of the molecular similarity, caffeine is sometimes incorporated into the genetic material. Radio-labeled caffeine was given to mice during gestation until delivery. Then the genetic material from the pups was extracted. Radioactivity was found in the genetic material, indicating that caffeine was actually incorporated into the genetic make up of the baby mice! Perhaps our coffee drinking habits for the last 100 years will be found to be the cause of the "diabetes explosion" we are seeing in our country. We advise all people to avoid caffeine until after the childbearing years are past. And then, of course, one is in the cancer age.

Question: What is the reason blood cholesterol and triglycerides go up in diabetes?

Answer: Diabetics do not metabolize cholesterol well, and it accumulates in the blood and tissues. For this reason diabetics are well advised to take a vegetarian diet to avoid all cholesterol. Sugar in the diet or in the blood raises the triglyceride level.

Metrecal, with sucrose used as its sweetening agent, was fed to humans for one week. The triglycerides rose during that week, and stayed elevated for over six months. A matched calorie load from fruits did not produce the rise in triglycerides.

Question: Is it essential that a diabetic stop smoking?

Answer: I recommend that patients with the hypoglycemic syndrome be so strict about tobacco that they even stay out of the sidestream of people who are smoking, at least at first. Any alkaloid that ends in *-ine* is likely to be a member of the toxic alkaloid group which is always damaging to the pancreas. Examples are nicotine, caffeine, theobromine, theophyllin, and purines (found in certain animal products). We had one patient whose blood sugar always fell below 50 after she smoked a cigarette unless she had just eaten.

Question: Condiments have little or no sugar; why must they be avoided?

Answer: The condiments must be left out of the diet as they irritate the stomach. Since gastrointestinal problems are prominent in initiating and perpetuating this type of metabolic affliction, anything that would irritate or in any way destroy the good tone of the gastrointestinal tract should not be allowed. All fermented products such as sauerkraut, kim chee, and cheeses should be avoided, except those cheeses made from agar, legumes, nuts, or soy products.

Question: How does one handle social occasions that interrupt a set mealtime pattern?

Answer: Many social problems must be dealt with during the course of a year. Society is arranged in a fashion that defies the natural order of things. As a result, the physiologic processes are not in harmony with common practices. To go against the rhythmic cycles of eating and sleeping is more or less fatiguing to the body. An example is the anti-physiological practice of eating most of one's food at night, but getting most of one's sleep in the morning hours. Such a practice is a reversal of the physiological order, as sleep is roughly twice as beneficial to one before midnight as that taken after midnight; food taken in the morning is far more beneficial than that taken at night. Individuals beset by temptations and handicapped by weaknesses must pray for assistance and wisdom to know how to discharge all of one's duties, including social obligations, both to self and to others. One must weigh all factors when a meal is far off schedule: How important are the social duties; how likely is the irregularity to cause symptoms; and how costly will be the physical discomforts and disabilities?

Question: If you are very far off schedule, should you skip the meal entirely, or should you eat late?

Answer: Many times it is better to skip. Some patients find that if they have eaten far off schedule they will not feel well for two or three days and may not regain control of the appetite for several weeks. With such a price to pay, it is often better just to skip the meal.

Question: Do men have hypoglycemia?

Answer: Oh, yes! In fact, it is not at all uncommon, particularly in professional men. It is just more commonly a woman's disorder. We had a lawyer, some years ago, who came in with a severe case of the hypoglycemic syndrome. He denied having a poor diet, in fact, he particularly disliked sweets. His wife agreed that he was unusually careful. Yet, when he filled out his dietary history form, we calculated at least nineteen teaspoons of sugar used the day before his examination! He was surprised. We recommend, for healthy people, three to five teaspoons as a maximum amount for daily use; but most would be better off with even less.

Question: How much time should elapse after eating before you lie down?

Answer: Preferably two hours or more. The reclining position causes the weight of the internal organs to press against the very large nerve trunks on each side of the spinal column which shuts off the mechanism that keeps the gastrointestinal tract active. Therefore, as long as there is undigested food in the intestine, it is better not to lie down. We recommend a two-meal plan consisting of a hearty breakfast comprising half or more of the daily intake, and lunch comprising the remainder. Supper, if taken at all, should be light, early, and no more than 10% of the daily food intake. A cup of hot or cold herb tea is best for supper.

If the patient will get on a program of regularity, not varying the mealtimes by so much as five minutes nor allowing as much as fifteen minutes alteration in the bedtime and rising time, and following the diet we have outlined, within about three to six months many of these patients will have organized their lives and houses again, gotten back into society, and will come into the office with a bright face saying: "I am a new person!" Occasionally the transformation occurs in one week.

Most people with the hypoglycemic syndrome are chronically dehydrated. They need plenty of water between meals, enough to keep the urine almost colorless. One should not drink close to the meal, as the digestive juices will become diluted and digestion will be delayed. In addition to plenty of water, the meals should contain an abundance of fruits and vegetables and few of the heavy protein or fat foods such as the legumes, nuts, and seeds. These foods tend to be dehydrating. Do not forget exercise; it lowers the blood cholesterol, promotes digestion, and normalizes the blood sugar. While walking, breathe deeply and maintain good posture.

CHAPTER SIXTEEN

Regular and Spare Diets

The Weight of the Vegetarian

Generally, vegetarians do not need to be concerned with being overweight. They can usually maintain normal weight without effort. Almost everybody loses a few pounds of weight immediately upon adopting the vegetarian diet, but shortly the weight stabilizes, and soon a few pounds are gained back if one wishes.

There is not yet a clear understanding of the proper amount of adipose tissue that a human being should have. Humans, as originally designed by the Creator, were of good judgment and perfect self-control. They consumed the proper quantity of food without deficiency or excess and maintained life processes between mealtimes at top performance. For this reason, it would seem that the accumulation of appreciable fat on the body is an adaptation to this imperfect world. Nevertheless, in the present state, fat serves several useful functions.

Function of Body Fat

1. Body padding to prevent injury over bones and sensitive organs.
2. Energy storage for use during periods of reduced food intake.
3. Insulation against heat loss and storage of body heat.
4. Temporary removal of toxins from the blood and storage of toxic substances, with subsequent gradual release for detoxification, including alcohol, certain drugs, and various chemicals such as foodstuffs and marijuana.
5. Temporary storage for several hours in the skin and subcutaneous tissue of sugar, salt, and other potentially harmful nutrients immediately after meals to keep the blood from getting too concentrated with these chemicals.

Nobody can tell another person how much food is needed for his own body metabolism. Even mothers have trouble deciding if a child is overeating. The proper balance of intake and expenditure by humans is not currently known by anyone, scientist or layman. For a group of twenty or more subjects with similar attributes and activities, the food intake can vary as much as twofold. While there is often good agreement between averages for two such groups, the discrepancies between individual intakes and expenditures is often very great. Some people, through some mechanism of adaptation, are able to be healthy and active on energy intakes which would be considered inadequate by presently accepted standards. On the other hand, subjects have been given large quantities of additional food with little or no increase in body weight. Some obese people, in contrast, can have a drastic reduction of food intake and still not lose weight rapidly.[239]

Ideal Weight

One way the average American can figure his ideal weight is by applying the following formula:

1. Allow one hundred pounds for the first five feet of height.
2. Add five pounds per inch thereafter for females, seven pounds per inch thereafter for males.
3. Between the ages of 15 and 25, subtract 10 pounds for age 15, 9 pounds for age 16, 8 pounds for age 17; diminishing one pound for each additional year to the age of 25. The formula cannot be used under age 15.

Example: An eighteen-year-old female may be 5' 2'' tall. Her average weight would be 100, plus ten pounds for her height. Because she is eighteen, subtract 7 pounds, giving a total of 103 pounds. By age 25, the average female of 5' 2" weighs 110 pounds.

Another method of figuring weight is useful for those who have any physical problem or chronic illness, as in diabetes, arthritis, and other conditions of less than optimum health. Multiply the height in inches by 3.5 for women; by 4.0 for men. Subtract 108 from the product for women; 128 if a man. Some individuals recognize that they fare better if they achieve the lowest weight compatible with normal strength. This figure will often be 10-20% below the average weight obtained by the first formula given above.

The question naturally arises whether one can obtain all the nutrients required if one takes a low calorie vegetarian diet. It has been carefully calculated that on any reasonable vegetarian diet of unrefined foods, one can obtain the minimum daily requirements of all nutrients (which often lists at least double the nutrient intake required to prevent deficiencies) on about 975 calories. Most people will lose weight on so few calories. It can be stated with confidence that weight reduction can be achieved on a vegetarian diet without inducing deficiencies of nutrients.

Dangers of Overweight

Overweight is a common condition which can shorten life. While a rare case is made worse by endocrine imbalance, it is not usually the primary cause of overweight. All cases of overweight are due to the intake of more calories than are burned up by the functioning of the body; in other words, eating more than the body can use. Remember, there are many who are not overweight (may even be skinny) who eat too much, but in their cases, the body reacts differently to the excess food. Rats have been tested by giving first ad lib diets, then providing 10% less food than that taken on the ad lib diet. The rats weigh more on the 10% restriction than on the ad lib diets. Further, the lifespan is greater on the 10% restriction diets. We can postulate, therefore, that we injure health and make digestion less efficient by overeating, regardless of the weight.

Obesity may be defined as a condition of being 25% above the average weight; 10% above average being considered simple overweight. The overweight individual is in danger for several reasons:

1. Vital functions of the heart, lungs, gastrointestinal tract, genital organs, and muscles are hindered because of crowding from too much fat.

2. The nervous system functions improperly because of reduced availability of proper glycogen stores, reduced oxygen-carrying capacity of the blood, and reduced ability to transport oxygen from the lungs to the brain. There is reduced transfer of oxygen of alveolar air to blood, because of fatty deposits in the microscopic alveolar septa of the lungs.

3. Only 60% of obese people reach the age of 60, compared to 90% of slender individuals.

4. Metabolic disorders related to overnutrition include gout, diabetes, hypercholesterolemia, hypertriglyceridemia, and hyperosomolarity. These conditions result in heavy or viscous blood because of the heavy materials or fat dissolved in the blood. The heart must work harder with each heartbeat to pump the blood around, increasing the likelihood of fatigue and degeneration. Secondarily, there is premature development of various degenerative diseases such as atherosclerosis, with all their attendant ills.

5. Physical disorders related to overweight include high blood pressure, arthritis, an increase in all gastrointestinal problems, an increase in menstrual problems, sterility, etc. It has been said that being overweight increases the likelihood of having all other diseases, including the antisocial diseases of suicide and murder.

6. Cancer is more common in the overweight. An indirect cancer problem the overweight must consider involves those who use sugar substitutes. The Food and Drug Administration determined in March 1977 that saccharin is a cancer-producing agent. The decision was based on a Canadian study and at least ten other studies in which saccharin produced cancer. In one study, the cancer was produced at doses as low as the equivalent of 1.6 bottles of diet soda per day.[240]

Help for the Overweight Person

Many will be helped by some of the following suggestions:

1. Eat a larger proportion of the low calorie foods: tomatoes, lettuce, eggplant, summer squash, greens, cabbage, cucumbers, sun-sweetened berries, cantaloupe, etc.

2. Eat very moderately of dried fruits, white and yellow potatoes, beans, rice and other whole grain cereals, macaroni, and other pastas, breads and pastries, winter squash, etc. However do not entirely omit any of the valuable foods.

3. As much as possible avoid entirely rich and refined foods, fats (margarine, mayonnaise, cooking oils and fats, and all fried foods), sugar, syrup, and honey. Each of these foods tends to promote uncontrollable cravings.

4. Eat plenty of dry, chewy foods and uncooked fruits and vegetables. Use little liquid with your meals. Take small bites. Eat slowly, chewing thoroughly. This will cause you to be satisfied with much less food. Most people moisten the mouth with some kind of beverage, which encourages quick swallowing of food before it has been properly relished in the mouth. Remember the counsel: Take small bites and chew to a cream before swallowing. Don't be in a hurry to swallow the food. The overweight person should not take beverages, but should take lots of water between meals to provide plenty of saliva for chewing. Most beverages add much more in the way of calories than of nutrients.

5. Get daily outdoor exercise in walking or gardening. Do not use the car when you have time to walk to your destination. Walking 20-30 minutes a day will go far in preserving health and in reducing weight for most people.

6. Eat little or no supper, taking perhaps a grapefruit, tomato, cereal coffee, or herb tea (without milk or sugar). Never eat anything between meals.

7. Skip one meal or all meals one or two days a week (no more as a rule). The objective is to train the habits to small meals, well chewed. The dependence should not be placed in fasts.

8. Keep busy on a pleasant, useful program.

9. Look for some good study material on the subject of self-control and study the subject daily. The following are some excellent selections for this purpose:

Romans 6—Sin has no more dominion over you

Romans 8—Set the mind on the things of the spirit

IICorinthians 10:4, 5—Bring the thoughts into subjection

Psalms 145:14-21—Satisfaction comes from the Lord

Psalms 141:3, 4—Set a guard over the mouth

The Ministry of Healing—Chapter "Helping the Tempted"

The Ministry of Healing—Chapter on "Working for the Intemperate"

The Ministry of Healing—Chapter "Mind Cure"

The Desire of Ages—Chapter "The Temptation"

Testimonies for the Church, Volume 3, pp. 491, 492

10. Remember, overeating is curable. It takes firm will action united with Divine help, and a struggle may be required before getting the victory. Do not get discouraged or try crash programs.

Diet control is certainly the answer to overweight. Listen to this good advice given to a person living around the turn of the century: "If you should ... come down to a more spare diet, which would take from you twenty-five or thirty pounds of your gross flesh, you would be much less liable to disease."[241]

The battle is severe, but through trust in Divine power, "every deficiency of character may be supplied, every defilement cleansed, every fault corrected, every excellence developed."[242] In fact, you may expect that your weak point may become your strong point.

Diets for Weight Reduction— Good and Bad

In order to get fat out of the fat cells and into the circulation where it can be used for energy, cyclic AMP is required. It is of interest that caffeine blocks the conversion of cyclic AMP to AMP, as does also theobromine from chocolate and theophylline from tea. Purines, resembling caffeine, come mainly from animal products, particularly meat. It is likely that both caffeine drinks and all animal products make the fat and glucose rise in the blood stream, thereby encouraging the storing of fat in the body. Too much niacin also inhibits the transformation of ATP (a high energy chemical) to cyclic AMP, and may also increase the likelihood of storing fat.

Both caloric intake and energy expenditure must be figured in determining a proper quantity of food to be taken. Following are several thoughts and sayings to illustrate this fact:

It has been said that if one eats a single peanut per day more than his actual caloric need, he can expect to store more that 3,500 calories, or about one pound, in a year. This pound is added in the form of fat. It has been shown that typists switching from a manual to an electric typewriter can add as much as two pounds of fat per year by the energy saved. These simple acts count up many pounds in a decade or two.

Energy Used for Different Activities by Young Adults
(Including basal metabolism and influence of food)

	Cal./Min
Sleep (basal)	1.0-1.2
Dressing, washing, etc.	3.0-4.0

Light indoor activities	
Lying at ease	1.4-1.5
Sitting at ease	1.5-1.6
Standing at ease	1.7-1.9
Sitting, writing	1.9-2.2
Sitting, playing cards, or musical instruments	2.0-2.6
Transportation	
Walking, 2 mph, level	
Weight, 100 lb.	2.6
140 lb.	2.9
180 lb.	3.5
Walking, 3.5 mph, level	
Weight, 100 lb.	3.6
140 lb.	4.6
180 lb.	5.4
Walking 3.5 mph, up, 10% incline,	
Weight, 155 lb.	8.9
Driving a car	2.8
Canoeing, 2.5 mph	3.0
4.0 mph	7.0
Horseback riding, walk	3.0
trot	8.0
Cycling, 5.5 mph	4.5
9.4 mph	7.0
Stair climbing	
Weight, 140 lb.	6.2
180 lb.	8.6
Walking on loose snow, level, 2.5 mph,	
180 lb. man, with 44 lb. pack	20.2
Work tasks	
Sweeping floors	1.7
Machine sewing	2.8
Scrubbing, kneeling	3.4
Ironing	4.2
Typing, 40 words/minute	
Manual typewriter	1.5
Electric typewriter	1.3
Gardening, weeding	4.4-5.6
digging	8.6
Ploughing with tractor	4.2
Light industry, printing, etc.	2.2-3.0
Carpentry tasks	2.4-9.1
Coal mining tasks	5.3-8.0
Recreation involving moderate exercise	
Playing with children	3.5
Archery	5.2
Tennis	7.0
Recreation involving hard exercise	
Swimming	5.0-11.0
Cross-country running	10.6

Climbing, light load and slope	10.7
heavy load and slope	13.2
Skiing, hard snow	
Level, 3.7 mph	9.9
Uphill, maximum speed	18.6

*Adapted from Passmore, R., and Durnin, J. V. G. A.: Human energy expenditure. Physiol. Rev., *35*:801, 1955.

"The only (reducing) diet anyone belongs on is the one he is going to be on the rest of his life." (An unidentified physician writing in a health journal of the last century).

A proper reducing diet eliminates all empty calories such as sugar, fat, alcohol, and anything made with them. Menus will emphasize three classes of simple foods prepared in a natural, yet tasty way: fruits, vegetables, and whole grains. If the individual can be persuaded to accept this diet and adapt his needs to it, he will find that his satisfaction with food is the most complete it has ever been, and that he can readily control his weight with this simple dietary. Breakfast should be whole grains and fruits; dinners should be whole grains and vegetables plus legumes. The overweight individual should painstakingly train himself to a two-meal plan, having all major meals finished by four in the afternoon. Food taken after 4:00 p.m. is more likely to be stored as fat. Supper should be omitted entirely, unless the weight begins to fall below the ideal.

Nothing is gained by having an overweight person eat a starvation diet. The weight loss should be approximately ten pounds maximum during the first week, and one or two pounds maximum during all subsequent weeks. Unless a person is taking quite a lot of exercise, if the weight loss exceeds two pounds per week, it can be assumed that the program will eventually fail. One-half pound per week is a good level of weight loss for simple overweight or obesity, not complicated by disease which might necessitate more rapid weight loss.

The individual must place himself permanently in a new lifestyle which is not to have a terminus at the end of the weight reduction period. Any diet that brings depletion of nutrients and starvation during its early period will promote overeating at a later time.

Some overweight people mistakenly believe bread and other high starch foods to be their downfall. It is usually *fats*, however, combined with too little exercise. The satiety (satisfaction) value of bread has been conclusively demonstrated. Refined carbohydrates are not as satisfying as those from the whole food. When a refined carbohydrate product of apples was given to volunteers, it was demonstrated that it was not as satisfying as the whole food. The same principle has been illustrated with grains. Whole wheat bread has been found to be more satisfying than white bread.[243]

Liquid reducing diets are poor, because the individual is not retrained to a new pattern of eating with its techniques of chewing properly, taking small bites, eating slowly, and dishing out a proper amount of the right type of food. These diets are also unsatisfactory, because they are usually imbalanced in some way, either too much protein, too little fiber, or too many of some vitamins and minerals, and absence of others.

Athletes are prone to develop overweight later in life. Some misconceptions promote this possibility. Protein needs are not increased by exercise. Overeating protein-rich foods during athletic training will not increase muscle mass, but may set a person up for a later problem with obesity. It should also be remembered in the training of athletes, that while carbohydrate loading increases endurance, it may also cause stiffness, angina type pain, electrocardiogram abnormalities, and possible long-term effects on heart and other muscles.[244]

The high protein diet is particularly harmful as it induces dehydration, puts a toxic load on the liver and kidneys, and causes an imbalance of the body's economy. Many deaths have been ascribed to certain liquid, high-protein, reducing diets. High protein diets bring a sense of false security because they "work" nicely; the heat of the specific dynamic action of protein increases calorie consumption by the body, excess water may be lost from tissue fluids rapidly, and only 58% of the protein molecule is available to be converted to glucose for fuel. The serious drawbacks come later, but are of such a catastrophic nature as to make all early victories empty.

The high or low carbohydrate diet is unacceptable, since any diet that depends on altering a major food substance by increasing or decreasing that substance in an unbalanced way will cause the diet to fail. Every individual needs a balanced diet, and the overweight person is no exception. The so-called 10-10-80 diet is probably closest to that which will bring the weight down and keep it down. The numbers represent the percentage of fat, protein, and complex carbohydrates in the diet—10% fat,

10% protein, and 80% carbohydrates. Although weight may be lost initially on an imbalanced diet, the diet cannot be maintained, but the maintenance diet for the overweight person must be maintained for decades.

The high fat diet does not provide sufficient minerals, vitamins, and proteins. It is to be condemned, because it tends to raise the blood fats. The high fat diet became a fad a few years ago, but was associated with several deaths from major heart attacks.

Common Errors in Eating That Lead to Overweight

It is those little faults, so common they are often unnoticed, that cause our downfall. In this category fall the faults of eating too much, or at wrong times. The mind becomes clouded by the toxic products that are the result of incomplete intestinal digestion. Thereby, we become separated from God, as He can commune with us only through the mind. When we have knowingly overeaten, we have demonstrated that we prefer the gifts above the fellowship of the Giver.

We should learn the difference between appetite and hunger. Appetite is given to us by a loving Creator to help us enjoy the food which we must have, and to make pleasant the duty to provide nourishment for the body. The basic need of the person, however, is not the enjoyment of food: the need is for nutrients. Appetite and the pleasure of eating encourage us to supply the need. Thoughts of food should not fill the mind. One may properly use appetite to assist in selections to fill the need. The need may be for raw food, for whole grains, for vegetables or for fruit. Appetite can help one to choose the kind of raw food, the type of grain, or the style of preparation. These needs have been established by the Creator, Who is willing to give us power to fill these needs. Through watchfulness and prayer, one may receive all of his needs, including the control of appetite.

In order for weight control to be successful, it must represent a permanent change in lifestyle. The old lifestyle has been demonstrated to produce overweight, and a change for a few weeks or months, followed by a return to the former lifestyle will be unsuccessful. The pressures of our modern society and the opportunities available for perverting the appetite induce many to follow a lifestyle that leads to overweight. Some factors are a hazard for one person, but no problem for another. The lifestyle must be evaluated and compelling attractions avoided The following items should be reviewed by every overweight person and corrections made as needed.

The overweight person generally does not understand the role of exercise in controlling the appetite. Vigorous exercise curbs the appetite. Mild exercise promotes appetite. Start the exercise program so gently that no sore muscles result, as soreness inhibits the willingness to exercise; to repair inflamed tissues costs something in biochemical activity that could trip the emotional balances in the wrong direction and cause discouragement.

It can be readily appreciated that taking large bites leads to stuffing. Combine with this habit rapid eating and poor chewing, and the stage is set for taking hundreds of extra calories in a short time. While it is unhealthful for anyone to take food only partly chewed, for the overweight person, the practice causes reduced satisfaction with food and a tendency to overeat.

A frequent corollary of eating no breakfast is eating between meals and taking heavy meals in the evening. Between meals eating is generally associated with inferior quality food, excessive work for the stomach which requires its rest between meals for top performance, and stuffing at night because of an all-gone feeling. The all-gone sensation is due to a type of fatigue of the digestive apparatus.

All of the following refined foods should be eliminated until proper weight is achieved: all oils and fatty foods (margarine, mayonnaise, fried foods, and cooking fats); sugar and other concentrated sweets; white foods such as macaroni, white flour products, spaghetti, and starch; food and juice concentrates, canned, frozen, and dry. These foods should never be taken generously, and some can be permanently eliminated as they are essentially empty calories.

Cravings are stimulated by a number of dietary practices, and by eliminating the practices cravings can be banished. Fermented articles of diet cause irritation of the nerves which lead to cravings: vinegar, mayonnaise, pickles, mustard, alcohol, cheese, and over-ripe fruit. Free salt use also leads to cravings. It is recommended that one use no more than one teaspoon of salt per day. Any drug that will stimulate the nerves will stimulate the appetite in susceptible people. This includes coffee, tea, colas, and chocolate. These beverages stimulate cravings. An irritant may cause the stomach to call attention to itself (See #8 on page 123 in the section "Weight Control Routine"). If it does, it may do so in a way that is mistaken for hunger. Much "binge"

eating has its origin here. One can train the habits so that one can stop eating when enough food has been taken.

One can develop habits which will enable one to know how much food to take on the plate and to stop dishing out at that point. A good practice is that of using a serving tray, placing on it all the food that will be consumed at that meal, and leaving the serving dishes in the kitchen to avoid the temptation of the presence of food on the table (a "little dab" left in the bowl is especially tempting).

The larger the variety of foods served at a meal the greater the tendency to overeat. Two or three dishes with bread are sufficient using adequate serving sizes; be realistic, as you cannot live merely on air or three carrot curls.

The proper use of the will always implies action. When a problem is recognized, decided steps must be taken promptly (even hurriedly) to remedy the problem. No half-hearted attempts will be successful, but to the contrary, actually invite temptation. There must be a cleaning out of the kitchen and freezer, a change of serving style, a serious study of nutritional needs, and a devotion to the principles learned.

Summary of Thought Errors Leading to Overweight

1. Allowing the appetite to accept as normal a large quantity of food.

2. Bingeing and repenting rather than changing and maintaining.

3. Taking too little exercise.

4. Eating too fast, chewing poorly, and taking bites that are too big.

5. Breakfast skipping or skimping.

6. Eating generously of refined foods.

7. Using fermented, putrified, or aged products.

8. Using salt freely.

9. Using caffeine-containing drinks and other stimulants.

10. Using stomach irritants.

11. Absence of a definite satiety level.

12. Large numbers of dishes of food served.

13. Lack of understanding of the proper use of the will power (action-remove oneself) and the steps necessary to resist temptation.

Weight Control Routine

A good, general step-by-step program for weight reduction can be adopted according to the following schedule:

1. Begin each week with a twenty-four to forty-hour fast.

2. Get regular meals and sleep. Hunger can be experienced on schedule, by habit. "Correct" sleep enables one to have energy to operate the actions needed in will power.

3. Get a good breakfast. Sample: 1-1¼ cups of a cooked cereal, two 100-calorie servings of fruit (one raw, one not raw), and one slice of whole grain bread. One fruit serving can be a fruit sauce such as apple or peach sauce made from blending unsweetened canned fruit. Use the fruit sauce on the cooked cereal instead of milk and sugar. Use no empty calories.

4. Eat a good lunch. Sample: About 250 calories of a main dish from the list given in the section on *Main Dishes*, 100 calories of a cooked vegetable. a raw vegetable in unspecified quantity (providing there is no dressing other than lemon or tomato juice), and less than 100 calories of a whole grain bread.

5. Take not a morsel between meals. Make this one of the principles of life.

6. Have some light exercise after meals; it promotes digestion. Never lie down after meals.

7. Get moderate exercise in the amount of one to five hours daily. Heavy exercise suppresses the appetite.

8. Avoid stomach irritants. Anything that irritates the stomach or nervous system acts as a stimulant to the appetite.

9. Avoid crashes and fads. Retrain yourself now in a new lifestyle which you expect to maintain forever with only minor variations.

10. Drink enough water between meals to keep the urine pale.

Main Dishes

From the list below, select one item per meal as a main dish. Most Americans use meat, dairy products, or eggs (or all three) for their selection of main dishes. The main dish should be a good source of B-vitamins and protein. It should furnish 200-300 calories per serving. Some individuals need more than one serving, but the overweight person usually does not. The overweight person will feel more satisfied on a purely vegetarian diet, as the bulk of the food taken is greater on the vegetarian diet.

Legumes	Certain Tubers
Beans	Potatoes, sweet and Irish
Peas	Carrots
Peanuts	Rutabagas
Lentils	Turnips
Garbanzos	Jerusalem artichokes
	Parsnips
	Beets

Grains	Leafy Vegetables
Corn	Asparagus
Rice	Broccoli
Wheat	Brussel sprouts
Oats	Cauliflower
Buckwheat	Collards
Millet	Greens of
Rye	common variety
Popcorn	
Barley	

Seeds	Other foods
Nuts	Winter squash
Sunflower	Pumpkin
Sesame	
Pumpkin	

The "leafy vegetables" group from the listing above can be used as a main dish when calories must be severely restricted, as they furnish an excellent quality protein, good mineral and vitamin content, but very few calories.

Eleven Aids to Prevent Overeating

1. Before the first bite, serve your plate fully with all you should eat. This is the time to count calories. Be realistic, but do not serve more than the proper amount.

2. Have a prayer of thanksgiving that the Creator and Owner of your body has supplied you, the custodian, with such an abundance and such delicious foods that properly caring for oneself is easy and pleasant. Then eat with enjoyment, forgetfulness, delicacy, and nicety.

3. As a discipline, do not clean the plate. Set aside a portion of something you enjoy to leave on the plate.

4. Slow your eating pace; take small bites, and chew thoroughly.

5. Plan several pauses during the meal. It is not best to prepare the next bite while still eating the last. If you have something in the mouth, make it a rule not to have something on your fork. You may even wish to put the fork down between bites.

6. Take no seconds of anything except raw or leafy foods, and even then there must be no seconds on dressings other than plain juice such as lemon or tomato as a wetting agent.

7. Excuse yourself promptly when finished eating, usually about 25 to 45 minutes if you have chewed your food well. Leave the table at this point, at least for a few minutes. If you brush your teeth during this absence, you will find it easier to refrain from eating when you rejoin the table conversation.

8. Suggest a walk or other mild exercise Use this as a social event after the meal to get away from the temptation to continue eating. If continued nibbling is a problem, simply cover everything with a table cloth and leave. You will have more resolve after the stomach fills with gastric juices and the appetite abates somewhat.

9. Always preplan what you will eat at restaurants and social gatherings, then stick to the plan. It is a good idea to drink eight to sixteen ounces of water 30-60 minutes before a meal or a social function. The cause of much apparent hunger is really thirst; not genuine hunger.

10. Do not look at or think of food on the table toward the end of the meal. Instead, place your mind resolutely on a preplanned activity. Overeating is a form of hypnotism. "Weakness, half heartedness, and indecision provoke the assaults of Satan; and those who permit these traits to grow will be borne helplessly down by the surging waves of temptation."[245] "I beseech you.. that ye present your bodies a *living sacrifice,* holy, acceptable unto God, which is your reasonable service. And be not conformed to this world: but be ye transformed by the renewing of your mind, that ye may prove what is that good, and acceptable, and perfect, will of God."[246]

11. Get in the habit of putting even ½ teaspoon of leftovers in the refrigerator. Eat nothing more after you have quit eating your meal. If necessary promise yourself that ½ teaspoonful at your next meal, to encourage strictness in keeping the rule. Remember, if the food is lost it is still cheaper than if you put it on as storage fat!

Causes of Cravings
(See also the chapter on Appetite Control)

There are several situations and certain foods which promote indefinite cravings. These sensations cause unrest and unfilled longing and sometimes result in irrational behavior. Alterations in the lifestyle can prevent much of this distressing sensation. To control cravings, start with revising the lifestyle and being strict with all health habits, a sort of "cold turkey" treatment. Start changes by eliminating the following causes of cravings:

Sugar and refined grains
Milk, all dairy products
Salty foods
Stomach irritants
Caffeine, nicotine, and other alkaloids
Overeating
Hot pepper, black or red
Eating too fast
Eating between meals
No set time or place for meals
Tension or interruption during meals
Failure to eat with dignity and form
Inadequate or dissatisfying work experience
Too little exercise
Dehydration (keep urine pale by sufficient water intake)
Spices (ginger, cinnamon, cloves, nutmeg)
Vinegar, and anything made with vinegar: pickles, mayonnaise, catsup, mustard, etc.
Foods from a fermenting process such as sauerkraut, cheese, soy sauce, and similar products.
Baking soda and baking powder products, including Ritz, Saltines, and all commercial cookies, doughnuts, and many other bakery items.
Caffeine, theophylline, and nicotine, coffee, tea, colas, and chocolate.

• Drinking with meals. Digestion and stomach emptying are both delayed. Beverages, soups, juices, and milks should all be used sparingly. Stagnation in the stomach is one of the commonest causes of ulcers and gastritis.

• Late evening meals. Undigested food in the stomach after retiring is a burden and usually spends several hours longer in clearing the stomach than food taken before about five o'clock.

• Eating too much. Most people could get by very well with one-half or two-thirds less than they presently consume.

• Chewing too little. Eating too fast. Bites too large (use ⅓ of a forkful or ⅓ of a spoonful).

• Foods rich in refined sugar, refined oils, vitamin and mineral preparations, or concentrated proteins such as heavy meat substitutes and dried milk products. The more concentrated the food, the more likely to irritate the stomach.

• Eating fruits and vegetables at the same meal. Foods that contain combinations of milk and eggs, milk and sugar, or eggs and sugar.

• Unripe or overripe fruit.

• Foods that are taken while they are too hot or too cold.

• Crowding meals closer together than five hours.

Sample Menu for Reducing Diet

Breakfast

Main dish: 1 cup cooked cereal or
⅓ cup of simple granola OR
2 slices of whole wheat bread
Fruits: 2 average servings of fruit, at least one of which is raw
Bread: ½ slice toast
Spread: 1½ teaspoons emulsified peanut butter OR
¾ teaspoon plain peanut butter

Use no milk or butter on the cereal, but eat cereal with a fruit sauce used as one of the fruit servings. Emulsify peanut butter by mixing equal quantities of peanut butter and water and stirring until it becomes the consistency of soft pudding.

Lunch

Main Dish: ⅔ cup main dish such as well-cooked dry beans OR
1 large burger
Cooked
vegetable: 100 calories of cooked vegetables
Raw
Vegetable: Raw dish (seconds permitted with lemon juice only)
Bread: 1 slice bread
Spread Small amount of spread if made without oil (See recipes in Eat for Strength, Oil Free Edition)
Supper: One or two cups of hot herb tea may be taken

Underweight

Underweight is treated with the same basic diet as for overweight individuals. The underweight person should eat plenty, but should not stuff himself. Stuffing is ineffectual, as most underweight persons can attest. Nor is it wise to burden the digestive organs with a mass of rich foods. Digestion is hindered and inefficient if rich foods are generously eaten. The same can be said for eating between meals. It is always a poor practice to eat between meals, as digestion and assimilation are hindered. For underweight persons, eating huge quantities and at unreasonable hours is always a mistake, as the digestive tract is already failing to digest and absorb sufficient amounts of the food eaten to maintain average weight. If poor health practices are put on as an added burden, even less efficient digestion may result.

A program of regular exercise, good meals served with gratitude, taking small bites, chewing thoroughly, and eating slowly will be the most effective program for an underweight person. "If one is thin, don't eat fast. If one is fat, don't eat: fast." This old jingle is still a good rule of thumb for thin people (and fat ones too!)

Sprouting

Sprouts fit very nicely into diets for the overweight. They are generally low in calories and high in nutrients. We should do all we can to promote the use of sprouts. During certain times of the year eating lettuce is somewhat like eating gold leaves. For a few cents, nourishing salad material can be grown by sprouting. Considering the ease, the economy, and the nutritional advantages of sprouting, it is surprising that it is only now catching on. In two to seven days, anyone can make sprouts by simply soaking fertile dried seeds.

Advantages of Sprouting. Seeds can be kept dry for many months or even years and still be suitable for sprouting. The sprouting process accomplishes biologically what grinding does through the use of physical means and heating does through chemical changes. The chemical bonds for long-term storage of nutrients are broken through the sprouting process, making them more easily available for use by the body. Additionally, there is the development of vitamins C, A, and B, and the development of chlorophyll. Sprouting increases the content of vitamins B-1, B-2, C, niacin, pantothenic acid, pyridoxine, biotin, and folic acid.[247]

Seeds to Be Sprouted. Any seed that will grow can be sprouted in a jar and used in cooking. A special favorite is alfalfa. Radish seeds, all the legumes (especially popular are lentils, soybeans, and mung beans), and many grains are suitable for sprouting. Lettuce, radishes, and similar plants that "go to seed" furnish good seeds for sprouting. Simply gather the seed heads from the garden and save the seeds until the need for sprouts arises.

Uses for Sprouts. In winter, when greens are in short supply and are expensive in the market, sprouts can be prepared in the kitchen for use at a very inexpensive price. One can do one's own organic gardening in the kitchen. This kind of gardening requires no weed killing and no mulching. With judicious planning, sprouts can always be ready for use.

Sprouts can be used separately with a little salad dressing such as soy mayonnaise, or may be used with other greens, tomatoes, celery, bell pepper, grated carrots, etc., as a tossed salad. Grated carrots tossed with sprouts make a very fine salad. A good way to grate carrots is by putting them through a juicer and then mixing the juice back with the pulp to make a very fine grated salad.

Sprouts may be added to soups at the moment of serving. A favorite way to serve a thick vegetable stew is to float a large handful of sprouts on the top, and drop a small amount of soy mayonnaise on the mound. Sprouts may be liquified in tomato juice or nut milk in the blender to make a delicious and nutritious beverage, using a sprinkle of salt. They may be sprinkled on potato or pumpkin pie for an unusual and crispy dessert. The use of sour soy cream or soyannaise on top of the dessert make a delightful blend of the sweet and sour. Sprouted wheat or sunflower seeds are good with fruits. Sprouts may be mixed in breads, whole or ground. Bean sprouts, used as a main dish, are very good in chow mein or burgers. Cooked lentil, garbanzo, or soybean sprouts are especially good prepared as a main dish, and served over rice. The cooking time is greatly reduced (to about 30 minutes) for difficult to cook beans such as garbanzos and soybeans. Many sprouts need only two or three minutes of steaming. Of course, any seed that can be eaten raw can be sprouted and eaten raw, such as sun-flower seed, peanuts, etc.

Method of Sprouting. The simplest method of preparing sprouts is that of using a half-gallon jar with a jar ring and a screen wire or piece of sterilized nylon hose. Three tablespoons of whole, unsprayed seed are placed in the half-gallon jar with a generous quantity of water to soak overnight. The next morning, the seeds are rinsed well through the wire screen or nylon. The jar is turned upside down to drain for a few seconds and then left with a kitchen towel covering the jar, as seeds sprout better in a dark place. The seeds should be rinsed twice daily through the screen wire (more frequently in summer to prevent development of undesirable acids). Gently distribute the seeds around the sides of the jar by turning and shaking. The wet seeds will adhere to the jar wall. Sprouts are ready for use when ¼ to ½ inch long. Alfalfa seeds can be allowed to develop up to one or two inches. After two days, place the jar in the sun for half an hour to develop the chlorophyll and vitamin A. Rinse in water to eliminate unfertile seeds and hulls.

CHAPTER SEVENTEEN

Advice for Pregnant Vegetarians

Diet

The diet during pregnancy should be generous, simple, and tasty. It should not be of an irritating or exciting quality. During pregnancy, more than at any other time, vegetables and fruits should assume a large part of the diet (along with whole grain breads and a few nuts). If ever there is a need for simplicity of diet and special care as to quality, it is in the prenatal period.

The animal products need not play any part in the diet, particularly if milk is replaced by generous quantities of greens, whole grains, and legumes. These are the very same foods the cow uses to produce milk. It should be kept in mind that the first rule in nutrition is a wide variety. Individual meals, however, should be kept simple, both the recipes for dishes and menus for the meals.

The appetite should not be allowed to run riot to indulge cravings. Some feel that any whim of a pregnant woman should be satisfied. Such is not the case. Her diet should be chosen from principle, not from impulse or perverted appetite. Her food intake should be carefully controlled to produce, during the nine months, a 25-40 pound weight gain, which is most conducive to the production of a healthy baby. In other countries where an emphasis is not placed on a girlish figure after pregnancy, babies are born healthier. It is good to have steady and ample gains week by week. Plenty of water should be taken, sufficient to keep the urine pale, so that the blood can be cleansed and the stools kept soft.

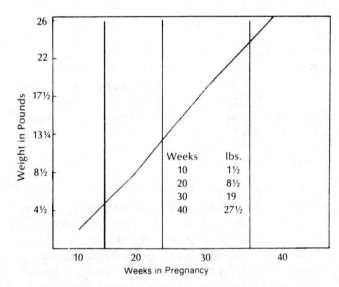

Weeks	lbs.
10	1½
20	8½
30	19
40	27½

Reasons for Maternal Weight Gain

Tissue	Weight (Pounds)
Fetus	7.5
Uterus	2.0
Placenta	1.5
Amniotic fluid	2.0
Blood volume	3.0
Extracellular fluid accretion	2.0
Breast tissue	1.0
Fat	9.0
Total	28.0

Certain Alkaloids are Toxic

Such items as caffeine, nicotine, and their members of the alkaloid group should be studiously avoided, as some have been found to be mutagenic. This means they have the capability of causing chromosome splitting, which can influence the growth of the baby. Any influence that might reduce the baby's IQ, by even a few points, should be carefully and meticulously avoided. Caffeine is found in coffee, tea, chocolate, colas, and some other soft drinks. Nicotine is found in tobacco. Theophylline and theobromine are found in tea and chocolate respectively.

Alcohol and Other Drugs

All poisonous drugs, foods containing toxic chemicals, and over the counter drugs should be faithfully omitted during pregnancy as at all other times. Most drugs can influence the growth of the baby, and such drugs as alcohol have been determined to cause below normal intelligence and physical development. It is wise to omit the use of any hormones except those that may be essential replacements, as in the case of insulin or thyroxin. Several of the manufactured hormones sometimes used as pregnancy tests or to try to maintain pregnancy in a threatened abortion have been found to cause birth defects.

Mental Attitude

The mental attitude of the mother during pregnancy is very important, as the baby can indeed be influenced by the mother's thoughts during pregnancy. She should encourage a constantly happy, cheerful, and contented disposition. Women have need of great patience before they are qualified to become mothers. If, before the birth of her child, she is self-indulgent, selfish, impatient, and exacting, these traits will be reflected in the disposition of the child. But, if she is temperate and self-denying, is kind, gentle, and unselfish, she may give her child these same precious traits of character.

She must not overwork. Most especially, she should not become overheated as by long hours spent in canning or baking, hot baths, or outdoor activities including sunbathing in the heat of the day. She should not be burdened with many stresses, and every attempt should be made to meet her physiological, psychological, and nutritional needs. The husband should be affable, courteous, kind and tender. He can help his wife avoid many physical ills and emotional and social difficulties. By his watchcare, many an illness can be kept away from his door (from his wife as well as from the children). The care given in the prenatal period determines the outcome of the pregnancy and the lifetime health of the baby far more than sophisticated equipment used in labor and delivery. Advances in knowledge of nutrition, exercise, fresh air, sunshine, regulation of habits, and the use of water have made it possible for the nine months of pregnancy to be a happy, healthy time, free from the hazards of yesteryear. Mothers and babies are healthier. It is largely because of the prenatal instructions, the good diet, the outdoor exercise, and the loose clothing that the life of the mother and that of the baby are healthier than before.

Exercise

The most neglected item in a prenatal program is usually that of exercise. Many other difficulties can be corrected by an adequate program of exercise. Some portion of each day should be spent in exercise out-of-doors. At first, spend one hour, and gradually increase the time spent until several hours are spent out-of-doors each day. The amount and quality of the blood that supplies the placenta are largely determined by the quality of the mother's physical activity. Exercise increases the blood perfusion to the placenta, thereby insuring a generous supply of oxygen, nutrients, and other growth chemicals to the baby. A proper rate of growth, not too much—not too little, is far more common in babies carried by mothers whose exercise is of a proper quantity and type.

An especially good type of exercise is that done on the hands and knees. Since the heaviest part of the baby is the back, to assume the hands and knees position allows the baby's back to drop to the front of the mother; the most favorable position for passage through the birth canal.

Keep a regular daily schedule, doing things at the same time each day. This will include weekends and holidays. Especially should bedtime, arising time, and meal times be regular, so that the circadian rhythm of the body can be as perfect as possible. Pregnancy is a timed condition, just as are the cycles of menstruation. For the proper automatic timing of each event in pregnancy, the lifestyle should be as regular as possible. Premature labor is to be prevented if at all possible, as premature babies are handicapped babies. Premature rupture of the membranes and premature labor are far less likely in women who refrain from the use of nicotine and caffeine, and who do not have marital relations in the last month of pregnancy.

Clothing

Not only should there never be a sense of chilliness during pregnancy, but the pregnant woman should frequently check her skin to be certain she does not have chilled extremities. Simply compare the temperature of the forehead with that of the backs of the arms, the wrists, ankles, knees, and sides of the thighs. They should all be of the same temperature, indicating a balanced circulation. The circulation to the placenta, and therefore the development of the baby, can be impeded by chilled extremities. Large blood vessels supply the limbs. Chilling causes them to become narrow and to carry less blood. The blood displaced from the limbs is available to congest the placenta and reduce the circulation. Slowed circulation in the extremities encourages the accumulation of toxic wastes, which are later thrown into the circulation on rewarming, to make the baby's blood impure. Tight bands across the abdomen or around any body part reduces circulation and should be avoided.

CHAPTER EIGHTEEN

Vegetarian Diet in Childhood

Generous Diet in Childhood

Since all human beings are composed of what they eat, the defects that show up in childhood, and later in adult life, are often due to the kind and quality of food eaten. This is especially true during the period of most rapid growth. Food must contain a generous number of nutritive factors (known and unknown) that the Creator provided for our needs, in as near their natural state as possible. Food that is whole, unrefined, and that has gone through the least processing is the best for growth and development.

Eating habits are not inherited, but are developed. The wise mother will take time and patience to teach the child good habits. Each meal-time should be approached with calm expectancy and patient understanding. There should be no hurry, no large bites, and no encouragement to eat faster or a larger quantity than in desired. There should be no force feeding. When the child indicates that he does not want a certain food in the meal, the mother should discipline *herself* to leave it off. If, however, the child sets up a pattern of omitting certain key foods, the mother should offer these foods alone at the first of the meal, while the child is the hungriest.

Breast Milk, Baby's First Food

Mother's milk is the perfect food for the infant. He needs no other food or beverage until he reaches six months of age. To introduce solid foods too early promotes the development of allergies in later life. Americans often insist that babies eat solid foods and take dairy milk long before their alimentary tracts are sufficiently developed to handle it properly. As a result, part of the chemicals in foods, unchanged by digestion, escape through the lining of the intestine, and get into the blood stream in an injurious form. The infant's "shock organs" become sensitized to the food, and ever thereafter, he is more likely to react with allergies. There is a widely circulated idea that adults who were breast-fed as infants have an average IQ about five points higher than those who were formula-fed. This statement is certainly believable from a nutritional basis, because of the presence of the amino acids taurine and cystine in mother's milk, which are believed by neurophysiologists to be specific nerve cell developers. Every encouragement and a herculean effort should be put forth to accomplish breast feeding. Nothing induces us to make a house call more urgently than does a serious threat to continuation of breast feeding.

Nutrient Content of Human and Cow's Milk

Nutrient	Human Milk	Cow's Milk
	(per 100 ml. of milk)	
Protein (gm.)	1.1	3.5
Vitamin A (I.U.)	240.0 (45)	140.0 (63)
Vitamin D (I.U.)	42.0	41.0
Vitamin E (I.U.)	0.56	0.13
Asorbic acid (mg.)	5.0	1.0
Folacin (mg.)	0.18	0.006
Niacin (mg. equiv.)	0.2 mg.	0.92
Riboflavin (mg.)	0.04	0.17
Thiamin (mg.)	0.01	0.03
Vitamin B-6 (mg.)	0.011	0.04
Vitamin B-12 (ugm.	-	0.4
Calcium (gm.)	0.033	0.118
Phosphorus (gm.)	0.014	0.093
Iodine (ug.)	-	35.0
Iron (mg.)	0.1	0.057
Potassium (mg.)	51.0	144.0
Magnesium (mg.)	4.0	13.0
Sodium (mg.)	16.0	50.0
Fat (gm.)	4.0	3.5
Lactose (gm.)	7.0	4.9
Casein (gm.)	0.4	2.8
Lactalbumin (gm.)	0.8-0.3	0.4

Breast Feeding Good for Mother and Child

Breast milk will be easier for your baby to digest. There will be less sour-smelling spit-up. Breast milk is always clean, warm, and your baby cannot catch an intestinal infection from it, nor be allergic to it. Breast-fed babies are protected against colds, allergies, diarrhea, and various infections. Sudden infant death syndrome (crib death) is almost unheard of in breast-fed babies; colic is rare. The nutrients are perfectly balanced for your baby, making it the ideal food for the baby. No other species of milk will perfectly fit the baby's needs. Infantile eczema, asthma, and other skin problems are much less with breast-feeding. Obesity is rare in breast-fed babies.

Breast-feeding stimulates the muscles of the uterus and helps it to return more readily to normal size and position. Breast-feeding is more economical from several standpoints, not the least of which is less medical care for the baby. Even one month of breast-feeding is worthwhile, but at least seven to fourteen months is best for the baby. The baby should be weaned directly from the breast to the table, not to a bottle. In breast-feeding mothers, family size is smaller, as breast-feeding often keeps one from ovulating, thus reducing fertility.

Breast-feeding is sometimes associated with problems which lead obstetricians and pediatricians alike to lose patience and slide into formula feeding. These problems, however, can almost always be overcome. We have had only one lady in seventeen years of supervising breast feeding that we judged to be unable to breast-feed. She had both nipples burned off in a fire that set her clothing on fire when she was in early childhood.

If you find breast-feeding to be uncomfortable, consult with a physician or a mother who has done breast-feeding. Do not forget that many people will be ready to suggest a formula when a problem develops. You must be ready to resist the suggestion regardless of the source, even your physician. There is a way around most problems, and the solution should be diligently sought.

Cold compresses to the breasts can cut down on too much milk production. Oatmeal gruel can increase milk production, as can exercise and certain herb teas. Cracked and tender nipples can be prevented by carefully cleansing the nipples before and after the baby nurses; before for the sake of the baby, and afterward for the sake of the mother. An enzyme in the saliva can cause the skin to become softened, cracked, or fissured. Breast size has nothing to do with how much milk one can produce. Milk is produced partly at the time of feeding. Large breasts simply have more fat tissue, but it is a glandular tissue that produces milk. The more vigorously the baby sucks, the bigger his milk supply becomes.

Specificity of the Milk of an Animal

The milk of a species is as specific for that animal as its coat or any other feature. Reason would dictate the desirability of giving the infant the particular milk fashioned by the Designer for the individual needs of the infant.

Species	Lifespan	Time to Double Birth Weight	Protein Content of Mother's Milk
Human	70 years	180 days	1.2%
Horse	25 years	180 days	1.2%
Cow	18 years	47 days	2.0%
Pig	10 years	14 days	5.9%
Cat	8 years	7 days	9.5%

Introducing Solid Foods

A small amount of solid food prepared for the baby from the family table may be introduced at six to eight months of age. With a fork or a blender, puree a small portion of food with fruit juice, mother's milk, vegetable broth, or water (determined by the plumpness of the baby). If possible, continue breast-feeding well into the second year of life, to supplement the food the baby receives from the table. If there is some unusual situation, such as illness, absence, or death of the mother, the feeding of pureed table foods may begin as early as four months. Up to that time banked human milk if available is the best substitute. Next to that is a formula. A very ripe banana is a good table food with which to start, as it is high in iron and easily digested.

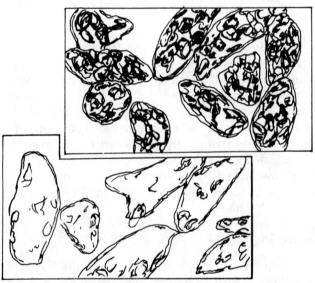

Unripe bananas contain starch, which turns into sugar as the fruit ripens. TOP, Starch granules are in all cells in the unripe stage. BOTTOM, Cells are free of starch granules in the fully ripe stage. The peel will be entirely yellow, tinged with brown. (Courtesy of the United Fruit Company.)

A new food should be offered, initially, once a day in small amounts (one to two teaspoons) for four or five days before introducing another new food. Give tiny bites on the bowl of a regular teaspoon. Baby spoons are often difficult to use; a regular spoon is much better. It is best for baby's digestion to give only one type of food at a meal. New foods are accepted best if blended thin and smooth. If the baby spits the food out, it does not mean that he does not like it, but that he has not yet learned how to swallow solids efficiently. It is wise to offer the same food several times, until baby becomes accustomed to it, and not to introduce a new food more often than every week.

Babies have different needs, and it is impossible to prescribe a given amount of food. The infant's appetite is usually the best index of the proper amount, but weight gain and development should also be carefully watched. Respect for his wishes will avoid many problems. If a definite dislike is shown for a food, skip it for awhile. Do not talk of the child's dislike of a food. Bring it back in small quantities later, without conflict or emphasis. As a general rule, it is not necessary to force feed a child. Family food dislikes are contagious and should not be made known to the infant. New foods are often best accepted when baby is hungry. Some prefer taking solid food before the milk, others afterward.

During the midportion of the first year, the infant will begin to drool and cut teeth. This is an indication that amylase is now being produced in the salivary glands, and it is soon time to offer starchy foods such as cereal and toast. After the meal pattern has been established, when he is not hungry at mealtime, he may refuse to eat. Let him go without anything, but let him understand he will get nothing to eat until the next regular meal. Some children will refuse to eat to get attention, and then eat enough between meals to take care of their needs. Be very strict in disciplining yourself to carry out this important health rule. The road to dyspepsia (poor digestion) begins with snacks. Do not allow the baby to become chubby. Overnourishment is at least as great a health hazard as undernourishment. Baby should double his birth weight in about six months. It is usually possible to establish a three-meal pattern by the age of one year, and a two meal pattern by the age of three years or earlier.

Three Essential Food Groups

The simple grains, fruits of the trees, and vegetables have all the nutritive properties necessary to make good blood. We can certainly say in this age of earth's history that: "... It is high time that we were educating ourselves to subsist upon fruits, grains, and vegetables.... A variety of simple dishes, perfectly healthful and nourishing, may be provided, aside from meat. Hearty men must have plenty of vegetables, fruits, and grains."[248]

Fruits. Nicely ripened banana, mashed fine and allowed to stand ten to fifteen minutes, is well-tolerated as an early fruit. Pureed prunes and apricots are usually well-tolerated and enjoyed. Apples should probably be left out of the baby's diet until after the first birthday, as many adults have sensitivities to apples which probably began very early in life. It is all right to use scraped raw apple to stop diarrhea. The pectin of apples takes up toxins and soothes the bowel. Many infants who are slow in accepting new foods seem to prefer fruits. Citrus fruits are often the cause of food sensitivities, and in all babies, should be introduced only after the first birthday. The same can be said of strawberries and tomatoes.

Select fruit which has not the faintest taint of spoilage. A basic recipe is as follows: ½ cup cubed fruit or vegetables (raw or cooked); ½ to 2 tablespoons of liquid (water, vegetable broth, or juice). Blend until smooth. A rubber spatula may be used to pull food down from the sides into the blender blades. Salt, sugar, flavorings, etc. are not needed.

Use only one food for a meal. Do not mix fruits and vegetables together, as they are more difficult to digest when presented at the same meal.

Vegetables. The yellow and green vegetables are moderately good sources of iron and vitamin B complex and are usually introduced somewhat after the midway point of the first year. A blender is a great convenience in preparing baby's food. He needs raw food combined with freshly cooked food. Opening a bottle or a can may be convenient, but it is not the best way to develop a healthy child. Some authorities are concerned about the addition of protein hydrolysates to baby foods, which may contain large quantities of the free acidic amino acids (glutamic, aspartic, cysteic acids). These substances may have a toxic effect on the brains of young animals, just as monosodium glutamate does.[249] The use of canned baby foods should be reserved for traveling, when it may be safer and more convenient than food kept unrefrigerated. You may puree the baby's food and freeze it in ice cube trays. Store food cubes in a plastic bag. One or two cubes makes a nice serving when thawed in a pyrex dish set it hot water. Carrots and beets are good for use in this manner.

Cereals. Any kind of whole grain cereal, well-cooked (liquified for infants) is very good in childhood. The ready-prepared cereals are inferior to your own thoroughly cooked brown rice, cracked wheat, unbolted grits, oatmeal, corn, millet, rye, buckwheat, and barley. Grains should have a long, slow cooking period, preferably one to three hours. Phytic acid, which ties up certain minerals, is destroyed by long cooking. The physical units of the grain are softened and prepared for better digestion with the long cooking period. It is likely that much of the food sensitivity manifested in

adults to grains could be avoided by attention to cooking time.

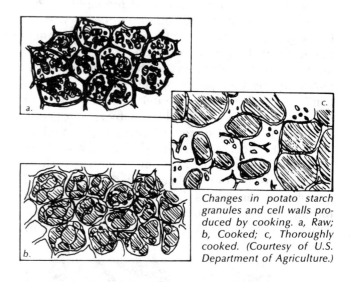

Changes in potato starch granules and cell walls produced by cooking. a, Raw; b, Cooked; c, Thoroughly cooked. (Courtesy of U.S. Department of Agriculture.)

Protein and Starch. Toward the end of the first year, when baby's chewing equipment is working, toast, baked potato (mixed with vegetable broth), pureed peas, and green limas can be added. Make your own melba toast from good quality whole grain breads. You may cut the bread slices into thin strips before drying. Dry the bread in the oven at 200-225 degrees Fahrenheit until entirely dry and hard. Melba toast is a good "teether" to promote eruption of teeth. Baby will enjoy holding the dried strips in his hand.

Weaning

Weaning is usually advisable when the infant is from ten to fourteen months old. However, to avoid the risk of dehydration, weaning should be postponed, if possible, during extremely hot weather. Teach the baby to drink water from a cup. He does not need to be put on a bottle. Upon weaning breast-fed infants, the bacterial flora of the intestinal tract gradually accumulates a larger population of coliform type germs, along with bacteroides. With the appearance of bacteroides, putrifactive processes begin resulting in a higher pH and an increase in ammonia and bacterial amines. These changes in the colon chemistry are followed by changes in the pattern of bile acids and free amino acids. The colon bacterial flora of bottle fed babies, even in the newborn period, is like the flora in the breast-fed infant after weaning. Such factors as traveling, infections, change of residence, and alterations in diet may upset the normal flora.

These bacteria can unload on man their unwanted metabolic products. While the intestinal flora probably shortens man's life expectancy, overall, their presence is believed to strengthen man's resistance to pathogenic microbes that could invade the bowel lining. The net effect, however, of the microflora is unfavorable to the host.

Before the infant is a year old he should be permitted to experiment with feeding himself. The ability to feed himself is an important step in the infant's development of self-reliance. It develops a sense of responsibility and has favorable repercussions in the years which folow. By the end of the second year, he should be largely responsible for his own feeding. The largest meal should be breakfast. Give dinner in the early or mid-afternoon. Supper can be omitted with good advantage to the digestion, the sleep, the temper, and the strength.

Since vitamin D is not a generous nutrient in the pure vegetarian diet, it is essential that the child get exposure to sunlight after weaning from the breast. A small daily exposure is adequate, probably the exposure of the face alone if the sunlight is bright. All persons responsible for the children's diets should read the vitamin section on pages 61-70.

Don'ts For Feeding a Child

1. Don't worry and fret over the amount of food an infant eats or refuses to eat. As a guide use growth and development, not the appetite to determine the amount of food a child should eat.

2. Don't use food as a reward or punishment.

3. Don't talk about a child's likes and dislikes in front of him. He "catches on" early in life.

4. It takes time and patience to develop good habits. Feed solid foods slowly; don't push them in fast in order to hurry through the meal.

5. Don't scold, discipline, or allow the intrusion of any unpleasantness at mealtime. Keep the home quiet and tranquil.

6. Don't allow the child to develop a taste for concentrated and refined foods. Never put sugar on cereal to induce him to eat it. Margarine is "empty calories" and is not needed on bread. Its only function is to make bread more palatable.

7. Don't allow a morsel to pass through the lips between meals, not even a sip of fruit juice.

8. Don't fall into the error of feeding too many dishes at a meal. The best rule is two or three dishes at a meal.

APPENDIX

Health Recovery Program

Rationale for Health Recovery Program

The health recovery diet is given to individuals who have symptoms of hypoglycemia, fatigue, allergies, headaches, depression, skin problems, digestive symptoms, and a host of other stressful disorders which are the product of modern society.

Caffeine is omitted from the diet because of the stimulation and tax on the pancreas. There has been a 300% increase in pancreatic cancer in the last century. We feel that the increased physical stress from concentrated foods, the poor chewing (which eliminates the beneficial effects of salivary amylase and causes a heavy load on the pancreas to produce such a heavy enzyme), the use of beverages containing methyl xanthines (coffee, tea, colas, and chocolate), and the great increase in between-meals eating are among the causes of the great increase in cancer of the pancreas.

We are now having what is called a diabetes explosion in the United States. Because of the massive increase in refined carbohydrates and refined sugars, the American population is peculiarly susceptible to overweight, heart disease, arthritis, depression, polycythemia (blood too rich), and diabetes. The health recovery program will assist in relief of these symptoms.

Eighty percent of overweight adults develop diabetes; probably 75 percent or more of these could be cured simply by following the Health Recovery Program. Follow the program for a full year before making any exceptions. Symptoms may clear rapidly, or very slowly over a year or more. Those who have a flat glucose tolerance curve can expect to be more resistant to treatment. After the year is up, gradually switch to a regular maintenance diet, while faithfully continuing the exercise, regularity, and other good health measures,

Physical Signs of Premature Aging Indicating Need for the Program

Acne	Overweight
Diabetes	Birth weight over 8 pounds
Arthritis	Heart rate over 80
Allergies	More than 5 fillings by age 20
Slow healing	More than 5 missing teeth by age 30
Cataracts	Rapid growth in early childhood
Tonsillectomy	Low resistance to disease with
Appendectomy	frequent colds, sore throats, boils,
Peptic ulcer	and skin and nail problems

Laboratory Reports Out of Ideal Range as Listed Below

Glucose 70-85	BUN below 15
Thyroid 4-12	Sodium below 140
Cholesterol 100 + age	WBC 3000 to 6000
Triglycerides below 100	Hemoglobin: Female 10.5-12.5
Uric acid below 5	Male 12.0-14.75

Uses of Diet

Use the Health Recovery Program Diet for physical symptoms and signs, or laboratory test results suggesting a kind of metabolic problem involving major nutrients.

Symptoms

Hay fever	Ringing in the ears
Unsteadiness on feet	Involuntary jumping or jerking
Diarrhea	Excessive cravings for food
Intestinal gas	Some kind of scalp symptoms (water
Heart palpitations	or ants crawling)
Headaches	Sensation of pressure in (or band
Dizziness	around the head)
Nervousness	Inability to dial a telephone number
Sleeplessness	without checking
Depression	Easily impatient or irritated
Shooting pains	Bizarre thoughts
Compulsions	Inability to organize work or
Fatigue	concentrate
Indigestion	A frequent sense of frustration
Constipation	

For menu suggestions see *Eat For Strength* cookbook. For the first year we recommend the oil-free diet.

Foods Allowed

Meats
A vegetarian diet is best. However, if meat and eggs are eaten, they should be overcooked to try to kill germs, and blotted to remove excess fat. Limit use in accordance with the recommendations of the American Heart Association to two to five times a week, except for objectionable meats such as pork, ham, bacon, sausage, hot dogs, hamburger, canned meat spreads, pressed meats, and canned composite meats such as Spam, which should all be permanently eliminated. (There are acceptable substitutes.)

Cheese
There are cheeses, butters, and sauces made from nuts, potatoes, carrots, tomatoes, onions or other vegetables and seasonings that provide delightful creams, spreads, and dips for vegetables, pastas and breads. Simple and inexpensive dishes can be made from appropriate recipes. See recommended cookbook.

High Protein Meat Substitutes
The products are best used as a temporary measure while making the change to the vegetarian diet. They are more healthful than meats, but not as good as the unconcentrated, unrefined foods from which these products were obtained. The meat substitutes are generally manufactured from soy beans and grains. It should be emphasized that all concentrated foods should be used sparingly, mainly as seasonings.

Breads
Use only whole grains. Two or three may be mixed for a single bread. Bread should be thoroughly cooked, and well masticated.

Cereals
Use only whole grains. Commercial cream of wheat is not a whole grain. If you like cream of wheat, substitute bulgar wheat or farina, or use the recipe in *EAT FOR STRENGTH* for cream of wheat using whole kernel wheat. You may also make cream of rice, cream of corn, or any whole grain. Some other easily prepared whole grain cereals are oatmeal, steel-cut oats, granola (without oil or honey), wheat cereals, buckwheat, barley, millet, brown rice, grits, or whole wheat macaroni. Soy spaghetti is also acceptable.

Vegetables
Vegetables may be used in liberal quantities. When used in the menu as a vegetable rather than as a main dish, the very starchy vegetables such as Irish potatoes, corn, spaghetti, macaroni, potatoes, or dried beans should be restricted to about 100 calorie portions. If corn, rice, spaghetti, macaroni, potatoes, or dried beans and peas are used as a main dish, a single serving should contain 250 to 300 calories. Very active persons, young men, and pregnant or lactating mothers may need seconds.

Milk Products
Milk products are not recommended. Milk sensitivity is the commonest form of food sensitivity in the United States. Many symptoms that have obscure or unknown causes have their origin in the use of milk. There is invariably a stomach problem in persons with the hypoglycemic syndrome. Leaving off milk will benefit some of these individuals more than they could believe.

Milk Substitutes
Recommended are nut milks, soy milk made from soybeans or flour (not commercial soy milks which are heavily sweetened), cheeses made from nuts, flours or vegetables; and sour and sweet creams made from special recipes. These milks may be used sparingly in cooking and in limited quantities with meals.

Miscellaneous
Green or black olives (not stuffed) and avocado (1/8 of a large one may be eaten.)

Nuts and Seeds
Use all kinds sparingly, as well as their butters (peanut butter, almond butter, sesame butter, etc.). Wash in cool water the shelled raw nuts, and sterilize them in the oven at 225° until dry. Raw nuts, sunflower, pumpkin, sesame seeds, and others may feel gummy while drying. Stirring occasionally hastens drying. Use nuts raw, or lightly roasted. Pumpkin seeds are said to be good for prostate problems.

Coffee and Tea Substitutes
All beverage herb teas are acceptable: lemon grass, gossip, lemon mint, etc. Postum, Caphag, Pero and other coffee substitutes are also acceptable, but some of this type of beverage have molasses or sugar beet residues in them. Check labels carefully. Remember that tea and coffee should be light drinks, not hearty and rich or nourishing. The only ingredient is water. All the rest is coloring, flavoring, or sweetening.

Artificial Sweeteners
It is best to learn to eat foods in their natural, unsweetened state as much as possible. One should cultivate the habit of leaving off sweeteners. If the risks are taken in using these substitutes, they should be used in small amounts, not more than the equivalent of three teaspoons of sugar daily.

Fruits
All fresh fruits may be used, and all fruits canned in water pack or natural juices. Bear in mind that fruit juices should be classed as refined foods, having had the fiber removed.

Foods to Avoid

Sugars:
White brown, or raw sugar; fructose, honey (for diabetics and hypoglycemics no type of honey can be used), syrups, jams, jellies, preserves, jello, etc.

Pastries:
Pies, cakes, any sweetened desserts, jello, which is only sweetened, colored, and flavored water with a small amount of gelatin (a highly refined protein). Learn to make your own pies and cakes healthfully from a good cookbook using no concentrated foods.

Cheese
Cheese is not the best food. The putrefactive process results in the production of amines, ammonia, irritating fatty acids (butyric, caproic, caprylic, etc.) and lactic acid. These are all waste products which cause irritation to nerves and gastrointestinal tract. Tyramine, one of the toxic amines produced in cheese may cause migraine headache. Certain of the amines can interact with the nitrates present in the stomach to form nitrosamine, a cancer-producing agent. An intolerance to lactose, the chief carbohydrate of cheese and milk, is probably the most common

food sensitivity in America. Rennet is used in the curdling of milk for cheese manufacture. Most rennet is obtained from the stomach lining of calves, kids, or pigs, and a very small percentage from vegetable sources.

Refined Grains

White bread, buns, melba toast, crackers and saltines, cakes, cookies, white macaroni, spaghetti, white rice, bolted corn meal, cream of wheat, and other refined grain products. Make your own whole grain melba toast and melba waffles. Crackers, cakes and cookies are unhealthful with baking soda or powder, eggs, milk, shortenings, flavorings, colorings and sugar. They can, however, be made healthfully. The whole grain pastas require a little more cooking, but with a bit of experience the cook handles these just as well as the white varieties.

Dry Cereals

Granola made with sugar, honey or oil; all boxed cereals

Sweet Fruits and Vegetables

All dried fruits (raisins, dates, figs, etc.) are concentrated foods. It is easy to overeat on them, overloading the body with too much food. Having overworked the digestive system most people will experience an "all gone" feeling before the next meal. This sensation which many do not understand results from a sort of fatigue of the digestive apparatus. Bananas, mangoes, watermelon (difficult for some to digest), and sweet potatoes should be avoided. Grapes if taken generously, may cause shakiness or weakness before the next meal.

Caffeine Drinks:

Coffee, tea, cola drinks, and chocolate (even Sanka and Decaff). Nicotine has been recognized as a cause of hypoglycemia. Tea and cocoa products cause constipation. All members of this group cause problems.

Soft Drinks:

All kinds, including Kool-Aid, bottled drinks, etc. Fruit juices may on occasion be used as part of the fluid in some recipes, but generally water is better. Fruit juices should not be taken regularly at meals in large quantities as they interfere with digestion, dump quickly into the blood stream, and displace other, more important foods.

Condiments

Spices have a number of evil influences on the body and nervous system. In India there is more cancer of the stomach, due to the heavy use of spices. Many spices are capable of causing distortion of mental functions and poor concentration. Vinegar, even the labeled apple cider vinegar, is irritating, both to the nervous system and to body tissues. Pickles may be prepared from a good recipe, being essentially canned cucumbers with lemon juice and salt. All products made with vinegar, relish, mustard, catsup, hot pepper sauce, commercial mayonnaise, and other products must be avoided.

Medicines Containing Caffeine:

Anacin, A.P.C., B.C., Caffergot, Cope, Coricidin, Dolor, Empirin Compound, Excedrin, Fiorinal, 4-Way Cold Tablets, Stanback, Trigesic, Vanquish, and others.

Some General Principles

Eat a substantial breakfast and lunch; supper, if eaten, should be only whole grains or fruit. We have found that the two meal plan allows the body the greatest opportunity for recovery from the heavy work of digestion. There should be at least five hours between meals. Do not vary mealtime by so much as a few minutes. Take no fluids with meals. Chew well. Blood sugar levels in rapid eaters fluctuate more widely than in those who eat slowly, and chew their food well. Expect that hypoglycemics may be nervous, irritable, and tend to get neurotic or self-centered, to brood over supposed ills, and to dwell on physical or emotional symptoms. Handle them with gentleness.

Many advise a "high protein" feeding between meals, with a bedtime snack, and even eating during the night. This practice is unphysiological and prolongs the problem. The pancreas has been overstimulated and requires rest for recovery. It should be stimulated only at certain specified intervals, so that it can regain its rhythmical pattern. Therefore, mealtimes should be very regular, with as little variation in time as possible, and *nothing* eaten between meals.

Caffeine and nicotine are potent stimulators of insulin production, and must be strictly avoided. Alcohol is highly injurious, a concentrated carbohydrate, a pancreatic stimulant, and a cellular poison. Even small amounts accelerate aging. To get "out of control" as a hypoglycemic does not mean that for a few hours he feels bad, and then all is well. The hypoglycemic may require some weeks to regain a sense of well-being after a short period of indiscretion. Some persons are highly sensitive to any transgression of health laws. And even if no ill effect is felt, the deterioration of the vital structures is proceeding more rapidly.

We advise that legumes (beans, peas, peanuts, etc.) and the whole grains such as rice, be used as a main dish as often as possible, rather than animal products. These simple and inexpensive foods are excellent sources of protein, and have the advantage that they do not raise the blood cholesterol or endanger the health from animal diseases. They also tend to have about one-third less calories than even the lean meats.

Drink enough water between meals to keep the urine almost colorless. For most people, this will average six to eight glasses a day. Drink water no closer than about fifteen minutes before meals, and wait about thirty minutes or more after meals. Generally the less fluid taken with meals the better. Much weakness and fatigue are due to compensatory water shifts, and the person is actually "wilted" even if no thirst is experienced.

Exercise is your best friend. Twenty minutes per day is *minimal*. One hour daily is better, but on certain days three to five hours may be needed. Do not get sunburned and do not make your muscles sore with too much exercise. Both of these are unhealthful. Gradually build to a good exercise level without ever developing sore muscles. Exercise helps keep your appetite under control, neutralizes stress, lowers blood cholesterol, promotes digestion, and normalizes blood sugar. Make it your daily companion. Breathe deeply while exercising and meditate on nature as you work out.

Do You Have the Hypoglycemic Syndrome?

1. Review the typical symptoms, signs, and laboratory findings given at the beginning of this section.

2. Typical lifestyle and pattern of surgical procedures. The typical person has an active social life, was "in everything" at school, and made good grades. Life has been rewarding until the present progression of symptoms has caused life to be unbearable.

3. The five or six hour glucose tolerance test usually shows typical abnormalities, but occasionally may not show them. No sugar should be spilled in the urine by normal kidneys in people who do not have diabetes. If the blood sugar is either very high or very low in a glucose tolerance test, suspect the hypoglycemic syndrome. The ideal range for all values except the thirty minute and one hour readings is between seventy and eighty-five. Any reading above or below this ideal may mean trouble ahead. This disease does not come on without warning. There are signals all along the way, from too rapid growth in infancy and childhood on through the dental caries and teenage depressions or rebellions, until finally the blood chemistries show up with higher than the ideal blood sugar and higher than ideal blood lipids (cholesterol 100 plus the age, and triglycerides around 100 or below).

This syndrome is properly called accelerated aging and is misnamed "hypoglycemia" which indicates a disorder of carbohydrate metabolism. This is not a one nutrient disorder, as there is *not a single nutrient uninvolved in this syndrome,* including vitamins, minerals, proteins, fats and water. Some feel that protein toxicity or fat overload are as important as carbohydrate sensitivity.

Books Recommended

HOME REMEDIES: HYDROTHERAPY, MASSAGE, CHARCOAL, AND OTHER SIMPLE TREATMENTS

EAT FOR STRENGTH cookbook, both regular and oil-free editions

For information regarding the above mentioned books by Agatha M. Thrash, M.D., write to: Health Education Materials Department, Yuchi Pines Institute, Route 1, Box 273, Seale, Alabama 36875.

Fat Free Diet

Do Not Eat	Can Eat
Meat	Wheat, bread, whole grains, cereal
Beef	grains (rice, macaroni, oats and oatmeal,
Chicken	millet, rye, corn, barley, wheat, buck-
Veal	wheat, and other pastas.)
Pork	Vegetables
	Fruits (no coconuts, olives, or avocados)
Cheeses	No-oil salad dressings
Eggs	Popcorn (hot air, microwave, covered
Salad oil	kettle without oil)
Butter/margarine	Butter buds
Milk and dairy products	Pudding (made with nut milk)
Boullion	Kidney beans
Ice cream	Sauces and butters made from cereals,
Pastries	fruits, vegetables, and combinations
Chocolate	Cheeses and milks made without oils
Nuts, peanuts, soybeans	(See *Eat For Strength*)
Fried foods	
Mayonnaise	
Peanut butter	

Drinks
Fruit juices
Water
Herb teas
Coffee and tea substitutes

Seasonings
Salt
Garlic salt or powder
Onion salt or powder
Lemon juice
Herbs (no spices)
Chopped onion, celery, parsley, cucumber, or tomato

Rationale for Fat-Free or Low Fat Diets

Fats are essential for proper functioning of the body, but fats added to foods are not necessary. Most foods contain some fats, including turnip greens, apples, cherries, grapes, squash, sweet potatoes, etc. Even when selecting a diet entirely free of added fats, one can be assured that if the foods are natural one will obtain sufficient numbers and quantities of fatty acids to supply all the body's requirements.

If one has severe arterial or coronary heart disease we may use a total oil-free diet, which restricts not only added fats but also most nuts, seeds, legumes, and high-fat fruits (olives and avocados); as well as all animal products (meat, milk, eggs, and cheese). We hope to accomplish by this diet the reduction of blood fats and subsequently the reduction of tissue fats. With this diet we can be certain that we are doing everything possible to encourage the reduction of fatty plaques inside the heart and arterial systems.

Certain diseases such as Raynaud's are characterized by a low oxygen supply to the tissues. Since fats in the blood cut down on tissue oxygen saturation, the attempt is made through diet to assist in oxygenation of the tissues. In these diseases, as well as in some milder cases of vascular disease, we may prescribe a "refined oil-free diet." It eliminates all refined oils, including margarine, mayonnaise, dairy butter, fried foods and cooking fats, but some nuts, seeds, legumes, and olives may be allowed.

Some other diseases are characterized by inflammation of tissues supplied by the rich capillary beds. In these disorders, plugging of small capillary beds by clusters of red blood cells may be a part of the cause of the disease. These red blood cell clusters are promoted by the ingestion of fats, alcohol, and other reducing substances, as the surfaces of the cells become sticky when these articles of diet are taken. Also, the manufacture of alcoholic substances in the gastro-intestinal tract promotes the formation of these clusters of cells that plug the small capillaries. Individuals with arthritis, inner or middle ear problems, infections, endocrine disorders (adrenals, thyroid, ovaries, etc.) and a number of other diseases will benefit from a low-fat natural diet free from animal products.

Fats are difficult to handle in the liver and a completely separate system for handling fats is provided through the lymphatic channels, a system of vessels that is capable of absorbing 60% or more of the fats we take in at meals. Were all the fat from a meal dumped into the bloodstream at one time it would overwhelm the liver and doubtless plug up all the rich capillary beds such as those around the adrenals, in the kidneys, around joints, and in many other areas. Our Divine Creator protected us against such a likelihood by making a separate system for the absorption of fats through the lacteals, which are lymphatic channels in the small bowel. In this way tissue oxygenation is not dangerously reduced by fatty meals in most persons. Nevertheless, individuals with diseases in tissues supplied by rich capillary beds should do their part to protect the body from the problems that too much fat imposes.

Rationale for Altering the Plant Steroids in the Diet

Contrary to the attitude of many physicians concerning diets, the level of steroidal compounds in the blood can be altered by the strict control of diet. If the diet is restrictive of all foods that contain plant steroids such as phystosterols, sitosterol, ergosterol, and others, a sufficient reduction in blood sterols can occur that withdrawal bleeding can be induced from the uterus in a certain percentage of women.

To control menstrual bleeding we often try a sterol-poor diet. For cancer of the breast we use a sterol-poor diet, as estrogenic-type compounds can stimulate certain breast cancers to develop and promote more rapid growth in them. In cancers of the prostate the reverse is true, and we give the foods that are high in plant sterols. For menopausal symptoms we do not use the artificial estrogenic compounds as these are known to increase the incidence of breast cancer in women from 12 to 35%, depending on the researcher reporting. Eating foods high in the natural plant sterols will control the unpleasant symptoms of the menopause in most women.

The Gluten-Free Diet

Certain grains such as wheat, rye, oats, and barley, and buckwheat (a seed) contain the protein called gluten. These patients may use rice, millet, and corn if they are not sensitive to these grains for other reasons than the presence of gluten.

Certain individuals are sensitive to gluten and suffer from gastro-intestinal symptoms, malabsorption, headaches, neurotic or psychotic symptoms, agitation and irritation, skin disorders, allergy symptoms, and a host of other problems. Patients with sprue and other gluten sensitivities will need to eliminate all foods containing gluten. Sufferers from Crohn's Disease (regional ileitis) should always be tried on a strict gluten-free diet, and many will experience considerable benefit.

The Nightshade-Free Diet

The nightshade family of plants is a very large one that includes several of our most useful vegetables, as well as some extremely poisonous herbs. The most common nightshade vegetables are tomatoes, potatoes, eggplant, and peppers. Even though they are excellent foods, they may create a problem for some people.

Dr. Norman Childers of Rutgers University has been experimenting for 20 years or more with the nightshade-free diet in individuals with arthritis and other forms of skeletal pain. It is his theory that the alkaloids naturally present in these foods such as solanine and tomatine cause sensitivities in certain individuals that cause not only long term joint pain, but eventually promote deformities in the joints because of overgrowth of the soft tissues or bone.

We have discovered many people whose arthritis was entirely cured in a matter of 4 or 5 weeks on a nightshade-free diet. Dr. Childers states that perhaps 10% of the population may be sensitive to nightshade alkaloids. He has found that 50 to 60% of arthritis sufferers may be substantially helped by omitting all nightshades.

The length of time for the nightshade-free diet should be approximately 3 months, during which time not a tiny speck of nightshades should be eaten. (Tobacco is also a nightshade, the alkaloid being nicotine.) Dr. Childers stresses the importance of avoiding even tiny amounts of these foods. If one puts the little finger in mashed potatoes, shakes it vigorously to remove as much as possible, then touches it to the tongue, in sensitive individuals even that tiny quantity can be enough to cause painful joints. The use of a little paprika (a pepper) dusted on as a garnish has also been enough to cause trouble in others. If one has conscientiously followed the diet for 3 months without appreciable benefit, he can generally assume that it will not help.

Rationale for the Salt-Free diet

A salt-free diet may be used for headaches, gynecologic problems, painful menstruation, high blood pressure, kidney disease, fluid retention or swelling in various areas, overweight, and other problems.

For thousands of years salt was used without paying attention to the fact that it might be harmful. In the last century we have come to understand the harmful effects of any nutrient when taken in concentrated form. As with sugar, fats, vitamins, other minerals, and refined proteins, we know that salt and the other minerals can damage the body in high concentration. A very high salt intake often begins in infancy with the feeding of cow's milk and high-salt baby foods. A salt craving can accompany a person throughout life. Many researchers believe that a highsalt concentration in the blood forces too much sodium (salt is sodium chloride) into heart muscle cells, weakening and damaging them years before a heart attack occurs.

We do not understand how salt injures the kidneys, but in some way a large quantity of salt increases the likelihood that the kidneys will be injured and participate in the elevation of blood pressure. Very likely there is a hereditary sensitivity to salt in most hypertensives.

In fluid retention or swellings, the presence of salt in the food can encourage fluid retention. One should bear in mind that wherever there is a grain of salt there will be a drop of water to hold it in proper solution.

A salt-poor or salt-free diet may be given for overweight since there is a great enhancement of flavor in foods with the addition of salt. For a person whose appetite for food is already far too keen, this kind of diet is very helpful. A salt-free diet promotes proper chewing and proper control of the appetite.

Certain individuals will have complete cessation of headaches when a salt-free diet is instituted. We assume that the influence of salt on arterioles and small arteries accounts for this effect. Individuals with hay fever may notice a similar benefit when going off salt.

It is easy to maintain an essentially salt-free diet at home if you observe a few simple rules:

1. Never add salt in preparation of food.
2. Never add salt at the table.
3. Do not use baked goods, crackers, or canned vegetables unless you have made them yourself without salt. Fresh and frozen vegetables are all right.
4. Most meats are high in salt; especially, never use processed meats, like hot dogs, salami, bologna, etc.
5. Eliminate all dairy products; they are all naturally high in salt.

By using onions, garlic, and other condiments and cooking herbs one can season food nicely without using salt. Remember that baking powder, baking soda, and monosodium glutamate all contain sodium and should be eliminated.

Principles Useful in Reducing

The most important dietary measure that can be taken for weight reduction is that of eliminating fats. Fats are used for the purpose of increasing palatability of foods. Since overweight individuals already enjoy their foods far too much, it is improper to increase the palatability of their foods by introducing fats, sugar, salt, enrichening agents, and other additives. All foods should be taken quite plain. Certain physicians believe that it is impossible for a person to become fat, or to remain fat, if all food taken is either plain fruit or vegetables. Since some foods require cooking to make all their nutrients available, a raw food diet should not be maintained for long periods of time. We do not recommend longer than one year of a totally raw food diet, and then only in very selected cases.

Dr. Fletcher, prominent in nutrition circles in the last century, said that it was impossible for one to be fat if one chewed one's food thoroughly. We recommend that persons who are overweight practice until they have perfected the art of eating slowly. This is no small task. Most individuals utterly fail at this simple matter. If small bites of food are introduced into the mouth and the food is chewed until there is no particle that can be made smaller, a great deal of satisfaction with that bite can be ob-

tained in the mouth. There is no satisfaction from food in the stomach, therefore the rational thing is to keep a small bite in the mouth as long as it is possible to do so.

Elimination of the evening meal is especially beneficial for weight control. Food is not needed during inactive periods in the evening, and puts a burden on the body at bedtime. During periods of inactivity, much less food is required for energy, and the extra food goes into the production of fat, cholesterol, and waste products.

Rationale for the Raw Food Diet

Because of the presence of enzymes in raw foods, some individuals feel they will benefit from using raw foods. Physiologists say, however, that the enzymes in raw foods are digested before they can be of any assistance to the individual who has eaten them. Nevertheless, the eating of raw foods does promote the production of enzymes within one's own gastrointestinal tract. In this way enzymes may be increased, but not from the raw fruits and vegetables themselves.

Grains and legumes should never be taken raw. There are toxic substances in both of them that are destroyed by heat. Sprouting may also eliminate most of these toxins.

Some individuals will lose weight better if they are placed on a raw diet. Since both weight reduction and a low protein diet are beneficial for malignancies, a raw diet may be used for a time in these individuals. Certain persons on a fasting routine may wish to break their fast with raw foods only as these may be more satisfying and easier to digest than cooked foods. Adult-onset diabetes, especially in the overweight, may be controlled much better on a diet that includes a high percentage of raw foods.

Since it is more difficult to obtain a balanced diet entirely from raw foods, and some people find it very difficult to take in enough calories to maintain a proper weight, we do not generally advise a raw diet over long periods of time.

Health Conditioning Centers in North America
(OCI, 1996)

Colonial Health & Education Center
18750 NE 63rd
Harrah, OK 73045
Phone: (405) 454-6653

Eden Valley Institute
6263 N. County Rd. #29
Loveland, CO 80538
Phone: (970) 667-0809

Living Springs Retreat
12 Living Springs Lane
Putnam Valley, NY 10579
Phone: (914) 526-2800

Poland Spring Health Institute, Inc.
226 Schellinger Road
Poland, ME 04274
Phone: (207) 998-2894

St. Helena Health Center
650 Sanitarium Rd.
Deer Park, CA 94576
Phone: (707) 963-6200 or
        (800) 358-9195

Silver Hills Guest House
R 2 Marble Lake Road
Lumby, BC V0E 2G0
Canada

Uchee Pines Institute
30 Uchee Pines Rd., #75
Seale, AL 36875
Phone: (334) 855-4764

Weimar Institute
P.O. Box 486
Weimar, CA 95736
Phone: (916) 637-4111 or
        (800) 525-9192

Wildwood Sanitarium, Inc.
P.O. Box 129
Wildwood, GA 30757
Phone: (706) 820-1493

Some Food Sources of Vitamin B-6

Brewer's yeast	2.50 mgm%
Sunflower seeds	1.25 mgm%
Wheat germ	1.15 mgm%
Soybeans	0.81 mgm%
Lentils	0.60 mgm%
Brown rice	0.55 mgm%
Chickpeas	0.54 mgm%
Green Vegetables	0.20 mgm%

Foods Rich in Potassium

Beverages

	mgm/100 ml or gm
Prune juice, canned	220
Tomato juice	21
Orange juice, fresh	205
Grapefruit juice, canned	200
Grape juice, canned	160
Pineapple juice, canned	160
Apricot juice	155

Vegetables

Soybeans	400
Red kidney beans	300
Carrots, diced, cooked	250
Lentils	200
Potato	200

Fruits

Peaches, raw, dried	900
Banana	200

Flour and Wheat

Wheat germ	700
Soy flour	600
Whole wheat bread	200

Food Sources of Zinc

Vegetables	mgm/100 ml or gm
Peas	4.0
Carrots	2.0
Beets	0.93
Cabbage	0.80
Watercress	0.56
Asparagus	0.32
Rutabaga	0.30
Lettuce	0.30
Potato	0.29
Corn	0.25
Tomato	0.24
Sweet potato	0.23
Cauliflower	0.23
Green beans	0.21
Turnip greens	0.21
Turnips	0.08

Nuts	
Whole nuts	3.42
Peanut butter	2.0

Breads	
Whole rye	1.34
Whole wheat	1.04
White	0.12

Fruits	
Dates	0.34
Banana	0.28
Pineapple	0.26
Red currants	0.20
Lemon	0.17
Prune juice	0.16
Cherries	0.15
Apricots	0.12
Orange juice	0.11
Grapefruit juice	0.10
Cantaloupe	0.09
Pears	0.08
Peaches	0.07
Apple juice	0.07

Cereals	
Wheat bran	14.0
Whole oatmeal	14.0
Wheat germ	13.3
Whole corn	2.5
Unpolished rice	1.5
White rice	0.5

Actual level in food crops depends on adequate zinc level in the soil. Many soils are deficient. In the case of cereals, the calcium phytate present in the products will prevent the absorption of zinc. Thus, the available zinc may be less.

Physical Signs of Human Zinc Deficiency

Erythematous and pustular dermatitis on neck, face, trunk, buttocks, legs, and around all body orifices
Alopecia — complete loss of hair
Diarrhea
Retardation of growth and sexual development
Amenorrhea or impotency
Lactose intolerance
Finger and toenail changes and infections
Dental caries
Conjunctivitis and photophobia — indirect gaze
High blood pressure

Increased susceptibility to infection
Impaired development of immune system
Gynecomastia — breast growth in males
Lassitude and muscle weakness
Behavior changes — disperceptions and confusion
This rare disease exemplifies many of the symptoms of zinc
   deficiency in man.
The disease responds dramatically to extra dietary zinc.

Sample Laboratory Report

Test	Ideal	Average Laboratory Reference Range
Chemistry:		
Calcium:		8.5 - 10.5 mg/dl
Inorganic Phosphate:		2.5 - 4.5 mg/dl
Glucose:	70 - 85	65 - 110 mg/dl
BUN:	7 - 15	10 - 20 mg/dl
Uric Acid:	Under 5	2.5 - 8.0 mg/dl
Cholesterol:	100 + age	150 - 300 mg/dl
Total Protein:		6.0 - 8.0 gm/dl
Albumin:		3.5 - 5.0 mg/dl
Total Bilirubin:		0.15 - 1.0 mg/dl
Alkaline Phosphatase:		30 - 115 mU ml
LDH:		100 - 225 mU/ml
SGOT:		7 - 40 mU/ml
Triglycerides:	Under 100	Up to 200 mg/dl
T-4:		4.5 - 12.0 ug/dl
HDL Cholesterol:		Less than 35: High risk of coronary artery disease.
		35 - 55: Intermediate risk of coronary artery disease.
		Greater than 55: Low risk of coronary artery disease

CBC AT SEA LEVEL		
RBC:	Female 3 to 4,000,000	4,200,000 to 5,400,000
	Male 4.2 to 5,000,000	4,700,000 to 6,100,000
WBC:	3800 - 5500	4,800 to 10,800
Hemoglobin:	Female 10.5 - 12.5	12 to 16
	Male 12.0 - 14.5	14 to 18
Hematocrit:	Female 32 - 38	37 - 47
	Male 35 - 43.5	42 - 52

BIBLIOGRAPHY

1. American Cookery, January, 1920
2. White, Phillip L. ScD. Let's Talk About Food. Today's Health 45:14, March, 1967
3. Rapid Growth, Short Life. Journal of the American Medical Association 171(4):461, September 26, 1969
4. Genesis 5:3-32
5. Genesis 9:3
6. Genesis 11:10-32, Genesis 25:7,8
7. Genesis 11:28
8. Genesis 11:10-32, Genesis 25:7
9. Psalm 90:10
10. Genesis 1:28
11. Government Report on Nutrition. PHASDA Facts, Third Quarter, 1977, page 3
12. More Cereals, Fruits, Vegetables, Less Fat, Sugar Needed in U.S. Diet. Nutrition Notes, Spring, 1977
13. Kline, O.L. Ph.D. Protein and Amino Acid Additions to Foods. American Journal of Public Health 50:1890-1894, December, 1960
14. Clarke, Gerald ....And Barking Up Another Three. Time 118 (23):80, December 7, 1981
15. Meat Versus Meatless Protein. Natural Health Bulletin, February 3, 1975, page 2
16. Unusual Facts about Plant Proteins. San Scripts 6(6), November-December, 1972
17. Sanchez, Albert, M.S. et al. Nutritive Value of Selected Proteins and Protein Combinations. American Journal of Clinical Nutrition 13(4):243-253, October, 1963
18. Toppenberg, Glenn. Vegetarian Diet. Journal of the American Medical Association 228:460, April 22, 1974
19. Hegsted, D.M. Ph.D. Protein Requirements of Adults. Journal of Laboratory and Clinical Medicine 31:261-284, 1946
20. Stahmann, Mark A. Agricultural Engineering 51(7):412, July 1970
21. Hegsted, D.M. et al. Journal of Laboratory and Clinical Medicine 31:261. 1946
22. Cerquira, Fry, and Conner. The Food and Nutrient Intake of the Tarahumara Indians of Mexico. American Journal of Clinical Nutrition 32:905-915, April, 1979
23. Ellis, Frey, R. et al. Incidence of Osteoporosis in Vegetarians and Omnivores. American Journal of Clinical Nutrition 25:555-558, June 1972
24. Agent in Diet Prolongs Life Span of Mice 44%. Medical Tribune, May 20, 1968, page 3
25. Intestinal Cancer May Be Increased by Meat Ammonia. Medical Tribune, September 20, 1972
26. Kuhnlein, U.R.S. et al. Mutagens in Feces from Vegetarians and Non-Vegetarians. Mutation Research 85:1-12, 1981
27. Hughes, James M. The Safety of Eating Shellfish. Journal of the American Medical Association 237:1980-1981, May 1977
28. Hand Infection in Butchers. Journal of the American Medical Association 203(10):180, March 4, 1968
29. Endurance of Vegetarians. Journal of the American Medical Association 36:1253
30. Letters. Nutrition Today, May-June, 1974, pages 33-34
31. Chen, Tung-tou and Chen-Pien Li. Resistance of Omnivorous and Vegetarian Rats Against Bacterial Infections. Chinese Journal of Physiology 4:59-64, 1930
32. Diet Changes Alter Stomach Flora. Journal of the American Medical Association 230(1):23, October 7, 1974
33. Drug Oxidation in Asian Vegetarians. The Lancet 2:151, July 19, 1980
34. Fat Malabsorption Is Associated with High-Fiber Diet. Internal Medicine News 12(16):29, September 1, 1979
35. High Level of Fat Excretion Seen with Vegetarian Diets. Family Practice News, 9(17):15, September 1, 1979
36. Carbohydrate Diet Wins Approval. News Bulletin from the 33rd Annual Convention and Scientific Assembly of the American Academy of Family Physicians 2(1): November, 1981
37. Steaks, Diet, and Drug Metabolism, Science News 110:376, December 11, 1976
38. Rose, G. Alan and E.J. Westbury. The Influence of Calcium Content of Water, Intake of Vegetables and Fruit and Of Other Food Factors Upon the Incidence of Renal Calculi. Urological Research 3:61-66, 1975
39. Eating Too Much Meat Considered Major Cause of Renal Stones. Internal Medicine News 12(9):1, 38, May 1, 1979
40. Corre, F., et al. Smoking and Leucocyte Counts. The Lancet 2:632-634, September 18, 1971
41. Pronounced Increase in Serum Creatinine Concentration After Eating Cooked Meat. British Medical Journal 1:1049-1050, April 21, 1979
42. Kay, K. Polybrominated biphenyls (PBB) Environmental Contamination in Michigan, 1973-1976. Environmental Research 13(1):74-93, 1977
43. Is There a Relationship Between Cancer of Cattle and Human Leukemia? Journal of Health and Healing 1(1):, Winter, 1981
44. Hepner, Gershon, W. Altered Bile Acid Metabolism in Vegetarians. American Journal of Digestive Diseases 20(10): 935-941, October, 1975
45. Aries, Vivienne C. The Effect of a Strict Vegetarian Diet on the Faecal Flora and Faecal Steroid Concentration. Journal of Pathology 103:54-56, January 1971
46. Dwyer, Johanna T. Mental Age and I.Q. of Predominantly Vegetarian Children. Journal of the American Dietetic Association 76:142-147, February, 1980
47. Cancer Research 41:3771-3773, September, 1981
48. Utt, Richard H. Predictive Medicine. Advent Review and Sabbath Herald, March 29, 1973, pages 1-9
49. How Farmers Make Food America's Best Buy. A.O. Harvestore Products, Inc. Arlington Heights, Il 60006, 1973
50. Robinson, Derek, M.D. Felis Domestica. New England Journal of Medicine 292(22):1184-5, May 29, 1975

51. Walton, Lewis R. et al. How You Can Live Six Extra Years. Santa Barbara, California: Woodbridge Press Publishing Company, 1981

52. MacLean, William G. Jr., M.D. and George Graham, M.D. Vegetarianism in Children. American Journal of Diseases of Children 134:513-519, May, 1980

53. White, Ellen Gould. Counsels on Diet and Foods, Takoma Park, Washington D.C.: Review and Herald Publishing Association, 1946, page 23

54. Ibid., page 138

55. Ibid., page 323

56. White, Ellen G. Healthful Living. Battle Creek, Michigan: Medical Missionary Board, 1897, page 91

57. White, Ellen Gould, Counsels on Diet and Foods, Takoma Park, Washington D.C.: Review and Herald Publishing Association, 1946, page 322

58. Ibid., page 356

59. Genesis 1:29

60. Genesis 6:4

61. Belson, Abby Avin, What You Eat Might Prevent Cancer—Or Cause It. Vogue, 167:235, March 1977

62. Diet and Longevity: The Link Confirmed. Science News 108(15):231, October 11, 1975

63. Cairns, John. The Cancer Problem. Scientific American 233(5):78, November, 1975

64. Campbell, T. Colin, The Web of Hunger. Natural History Magazine 90(5):12-16, May, 1981

65. Ibid.

66. Exodus 15, 16

67. Malachi 4

68. Exodus 16:15-35

69. I Kings 17:7-16

70. I Kings 19:6

71. Matthew 17:10-13

72. Revelation 13:17

73. Exodus 23:25

74. Deuteronomy 7:15

75. Psalms 106:14, 15

76. Numbers 13:33

77. Psalm 106:15

78. Psalm 105:37

79. White, Ellen Gould. Counsels on Diet and Foods. Takoma Park, Washington D.C.: Review and Herald Publishing Association, 1946, page 50

80. Ibid., page 112

81. Ibid., page 50

82. Ibid., page 483

83. Ibid., page 328

84. Ibid., page 91

85. Can A Vegetarian Be Well Nourished? Journal of the American Medical Association. 233(8):898, August 25, 1975

86. Ibid

87. The Cereal Marathon. Science News 119:103, February 14, 1981

88. Study Finds Academy Somes 'Subverted by Special Interests'. Science News 103(18):287, May 5, 1973

89. Silverglade, Minna, R.D. Organic Food. Journal of the American Medical Association 231:25, January 6, 1975

90. Isaiah 51:6

91. Genesis 8:22

92. Highland, Joseph and Marcia Fine. Malignant Neglect. New York: Alfred Knopf, 1979, page 218

93. White, Ellen Gould. Counsels on Diet and Foods. Takoma Park, Washington, D.C.: Review and Herald Publishing Association, 1946, page 309

94. The Deadliest Poison. Nutrition Today, 10(5-6):4-9, September-October, November-December, 1975

95. White, Ellen G. Ministry of Healing. Mountain View, California: Pacific Press Publishing Association, 1909, page 303

96. Proverbs 25:27

97. Proverbs 25:16

98. Ershoff, Benjamin H, PhD., M.P.H. Antitoxic Effects of Plant Fiber. American Journal of Clinical Nutrition 27:1395-1398, December, 1974

99. White, Ellen Gould. Ministry of Healing, Mountain View, California: Pacific Press Publishing Association, 1909, page 301

100. White, Ellen Gould. Counsels on Diet and Foods. Takoma Park, Washington D.C.: Review and Herald Publishing Association, 1946, page 110

101. Maruhama, Yoshisuke et al. Hasty Eating as a Cause of Unstable Blood Glucose in Patients with Maturity Onset Diabetes. Tohoku Journal of Experimental Medicine 130: 411-412, 1980

102. Selective Phospholipid Absorption and Atherosclerosis. Science 204:506-508, 1979

103. Quigley, J.P. PhD. Motor Physiology of the Stomach, the Pylorus and the Duodenum. Archives of Surgery 44:414-437, 1942

104. Newberry, P.D. Unsaturated Fat and Cancer. The Lancet 2:323, August 7, 1971

105. Controversies in Nutrition. Medical World News, August 22, 1977, pages 45-46

106. Goodhart, Robert S. and Maurice E. Shils. Modern Nutrition in Health and Disease. Sixth Edition, Philadelphia: Lea and Febiger, 1980, page 135

107. Campbell, T. Colin. The Web of Hunger, Natural History Magazine 90(5):12-16, May, 1981

108 Weihrauch, John L. and John M. Gardner, PhD. Sterol Content of Foods of Plant Origin, Journal of the American Dietetic Association 73:39-47, July, 1978

109. Nuzum, C. Thomas and Phillip J. Snodgrass. Urea Cycle Enzyme Adaptation to Dietary Protein in Primates. Science 172:1042-1043, June 4, 1971

110. Waterlow, J.C., M.D. Observation on the Mechanism of Adaptation to Low Protein Diets. The Lancet 2:1091-1097, November 23, 1968

111. Tepperman, Jay and Helen M. Tepperman. Gluconeogenesis, Lipogenesis, and the Sherringtonian Metaphor. Federation Proceedings 29:1284-1293, May-June, 1970

112. Munro, Hamish N. Metabolic Regulation in Relation to Cell Development. Federation Proceedings 29:1490, 1970

113. Muiruri, Kathleen L. and Gilbert A. Leveille. Metabolic Adaptations in Meal-Fed Rats: Effects of Increased Feeding Frequency or Ad Libitum Feeding in Rats Previously Adapted to a Single Daily Meal. Journal of Nutrition 100: 450, 1970

114. Intestinal Cancer May be Increased by Meat Ammonia. Medical Tribune, September 20, 1972

115. Adverse Effects Cited in Diets High in Protein. Medical Tribune, May 9, 1973

116. Unusual Facts About Plant Protein. San Scripts 6(6), November-December, 1972

117. Bogert, L. Jean Ph. D. et al. Nutrition and Physical Fitness. Eighth ed. Philadelphia: W.B. Saunders Company, 1966

118. Wallis, Allan D., M.D. Dietary Eggs and Rheumatic Fever. American Journal of Medical Science 227:167-170, February, 1954

119. Schauss, Alexander. Diet, Crime and Delinquency. Berkeley, California: Parker House, 1981

120. Kleiner, Israel S. Human Biochemistry. St. Louis, C.V. Mosby, Co. 1948, pages 222, 223

121. Wohl, Michael and Robert Goodhart. Modern Nutrition in Health and Disease, Fourth Ed. Philadelphia: Lea and Febiger, 1968

122. Beta-Endorphin: The Body's Thermostat? Science News 114(3):38, July 15, 1978

123. Campbell, T. Colin. The Web of Hunger. Natural History Magazine 90(5):12-16, May, 1981

124. White, Ellen Gould. Counsels on Diet and Foods. Takoma Park, Washington D.C.; Review and Herald Publishing Association, 1946, page 107

125. Yagi, Noriko and Yorshinori Itokawa. Cleavage of Thiamine by Chlorine in Tap Water. Journal of Nutritional Sciences and Vitaminology 24(4):281-287, 1979

126. Cheraskin, E., M.D. Protein-Nicotinic Acid Consumption and Early Psychologic Change. Mental Hygiene 53:624-626, 1968

127. Dent, C.E. et al. Effect of Chapattis and Ultraviolet Irradiation on Nutritional Rickets in an Indian Immigrant. The Lancet 1:1282-1284, June 9, 1973

128. Corrigan, James J. M.D. and Frank I. Marcus, M.D. Coagulopathy Associated With Vitamin E Ingestion. Journal of the American Medical Association 230:1300-1301, December 2, 1974

129. Horwitt, M.K. Vitamin E: A Reexamination. American Journal of Clinical Nutrition 29:569-578, 1976

130. Howard, Rosanne Beatrice and Nancie Harvey Herbold. Nutrition in Clinical Care. New York: McGraw-Hill, 1979

131. Burtin, B.T. PhD. Editor. The Heinz Handbook of Nutrition. New York: McGraw-Hill Book Co. 1965, page 111

132. Sebrell, W.H. Jr. and Robert S. Harris. The Vitamins, Volume 1, New York: Academic Press, 1954

133. Wokes, Frank. Human Dietary Deficiency of Vitamin B-12. American Journal of Clinical Nutrition 3(5):375-382, September-October, 1955

134. Leung, Albert. Encyclopedia of Common Natural Ingredients. New York: John Wiley, 1980, p. 458

135. Gyorgy, Paul and Pearson, Win. The Vitamins. Second Edition, Volume 2. New York: Academic Press, 1967, p. 8

136. Baker, S.J. and E.M. Demaeyer. Nutritional Anemia: Its Understanding and Control with Special Reference to the Work of the World Health Organization. American Journal of Clinical Nutrition 32:368-417, 1979

137. Bergevin, Patrick R. M.D. and Johannes Blom, M.D. Pernicious Anemia Terminating in Acute Myeloblastic Leukemia. Southern Medical Journal 69:110, January, 1976

138. Chauvergne, J. The Risk of Administering Vitamin B-12 to Cancer Patients. Semaine des Hospiteaux Paris 46:2170-2174, July 10, 1970

139. Igarai, Tadashi. Serum Vitamin B-12 Levels of Patients with Rheumatoid Arthritis. Tohoku Journal of Experimental Medicine 125(3):287-301, 1978

140. Herbert, Victor. Nutritional Requirements for Vitamin B-12 and Folic Acid. American Journal of Clinical Nutrition 21:743-752, 1968

141. Vitamin B-12, Methianine and Fat. Nutrition Reviews 18:110-112, April, 1960

142. Dryden, L.P. and A.M. Hartman. Vitamin B-12 Deficiency in the Rat Fed High Protein Rations. Journal of Nutrition 101:579-587, May, 1971

143. Siddons, R.C. The Experimental Production of B-12 Deficiency in the Baboon (Papio cynocephalus). A 2 Year Study. British Journal of Nutrition 32:219-228, 1974

144. Vegetarians Offer MD Food for Thought. Medical World News, September 14, 1962, page 33

145. Dastur, D.K. Effect of Vegetarianism and Smoking on Vitamin B-12, Thiocyanate and Folate Levels in the Blood of Normal Subjects. British Medical Journal 2:260-263, July 29, 1972

146. Linnell, J.C. Effects of Smoking on Metabolism and Excretion of Vitamin B-12. British Medical Journal 1(5599), April 27, 1968

147. Johnson, P.A. Cyanocobalamin. South African Medical Journal 49(33):1331, August 2, 1975

148. Duke, W.J.C. et al. Bacterial Synthesis of Vitamin B-12 in the Alimentary Tract. The Lancet 1:486-488, March 18, 1950

149. Contribution of the Microflora of the Small Intestine to the Vitamin B-12 Nutriture of Man. Nutrition Reviews 38(8):274-275, August, 1980

150. Albert, M.J. et al. Vitamin B-12 Synthesis by Human Small Intestinal Bacteria. Nature 283:781-782, February 21, 1980

151. Vegetarian and Vegan Sources of Vitamin B-12. Newsletter of The Vegetarian Society of the United Kingdom, Ltd. August, 1977

152. Shinton, N.K. and A.K. Singh. Vitamin B-12 Absorption by Inhalation. British Journal of Haematology 12:75-79, January, 1967

153. Armstrong, B.K. Absorption of Vitamin B-12 from the Human Colon. American Journal of Clinical Nutrition 21(4): 298-299, April, 1968

154. Dryden, L.P. and A.M. Hartman. Vitamin B-12 Deficiency in the Rat Fed High Protein Rations

155. Parker, Bruce C. Rain as a Source of Vitamin B-12. Nature 219:617-18, August 10, 1968

156. Jathar, V.S. Vitamin B-12-Like Activity in Leafy Vegetables. Indian Journal of Biochemistry and Biophysics 2:71-73, March, 1974

157. Gyorgy, Paul and Win Pearson. The Vitamins. Second Edition, Volume 2, New York: Academic Press, 1967, page 8

158. New Vitamin, or Just a Cousin? Medical World News, May 11, 1962, page 55

159. Herbert, Victor, M.D. J.D. and Elizabeth Jacob, M.D. Destruction of Vitamin B-12 by Ascorbic Acid. Journal of the American Medical Association 230:241-242, October 14, 1974

160. Hines, John D. M.D. Ascorbic Acid and Vitamin B-12 Deficiency. Journal of the American Medical Association 234(1):24, October 6, 1975

161. Hogencamp, H.P.C. The Interaction Between Vitamin B-12 Vitamin C. Americal Journal of Clinical Nutrition 33:1-3, January, 1980

162. Harmful B-12 Breakdown Products in Multivitamins? Medical World News, September 28, 1981, Pages 12,13

163. Doscherholmen, A. et al. Inhibitory Effect of Eggs on Vitamin B-12 Asorption. British Journal of Haematology 33:261-272, 1976

164. Dietary Fiber and Vitamin B-12 Balance. Nutrition Reviews 37(4):116-118, April, 1979

165. Brin, Myron, Ph.D. Drug-Vitamin Interrelationships. Nutrition and the M.D. 3(1):116-118, April, 1979

166. Choudhry, V.P. Vitamin B-12 Deficiency in Infancy Associated with Lactose Intolerance. Indian Journal of Pediatrics 39: 267-269, August, 1972

167. Ford, M.J. Megaloblastic Anemia in a Vegetarian. British Journal of Clinical Practice 34(7):222, July, 1980

168. Bailey, M.J. et al. Preoperative Haemoglobin as Predictor of Outcome of Diabetic Amputations. The Lancet 2:168-170, July 28, 1979

169. Garn, Stanley Ph.D. et al. Hematological Status and Pregnancy Outcomes. American Journal of Clinical Nutrition 34(1):115-117, January, 1981

170. Gleeson, M.H. and P.S. Graves. Complications of Dietary Deficiency of Vitamin B-12 in Young Caucasians. Postgraduate Medical Journal 50:462-466, July, 1974

171. Megaloblastic Anaemia in Indian Immigrants. The Lancet 1:575, March 11, 1972

172. Ibid

173. Wokes, Frank, Ph.D. Human Dietary Deficiency of Vitamin B-12. American Journal of Clinical Nutrition 3(5):375-382, September-October, 1955

174. Sanders, T.A.B. and F.R. Ellis. Haematological Studies in Vegans. British Journal of Nutrition 40(1):9-15, July, 1978

175. Hyperpigmentation in Pernicious Anemia. Nutrition Reviews 37:137-138, May, 1979

176. Genetic Factors and Pernicious Anemia. British Medical Journal 1:78, January 9, 1965

177. Fleming. A.F. M.D. Serum Vitamin B-12 Levels and Vitamin B-12 Binding Proteins of Serum and Saliva of Healthy Nigerians and Europeans. American Journal of Clinical Nutrition 31:1732-1738, 1978

178. Azen, Edwin A. and Carter Denniston. Genetic Polymorphism of Vitamin B-12 Binding (R) Proteins of Human Saliva Detected by Isoelectric Focusing. Biochemical Genetics 12(9-10):909-920, October, 1979

179. Adams, J.F. et al. Factors Affecting the Absorption of Vitamin B-12. Clinical Science 42:233-250, 1972

180. White, Ellen Gould. Counsels on Diet and Foods, Takoma Park, Washington D.C. Review and Herald Publishing Association, 1946, Page 275

181. Calcium Retention of Young Adult Males as Affected by Level of Protein and of Calcium Intake. Transactions of the New York Academy of Science 36:333-340, 1974

182. Howard, Rosanne Beatrice and Nancie Harvey Herbold. Nutrition in Clinical Care. New York: McGraw-Hill, Inc. 1978

183. Iengar, N.G.C. and Y.V.S. Rau. Green Leafy Vegetables as Sources of Calcium. Annals of Biochemistry and Experimental Medicine 12:41-52, 1952

184. Walker, A.R.P. and B.F. Walker. Effect of Wholemeal and White Bread on Iron Absorption. British Medical Journal 2:771-772, September 17, 1977

185. Walker, A.R.P. Cereals, Phytic Acid and Calcification. The Lancet 2:244-248, August 11, 1951

186. Bhaskaram, C. and Vinodini Reddy. Role of Dietary Phytate in the Aetiology of Nutritional Rickets. Indian Journal of Medical Research 69:265-270, February, 1979

187. Toma, R.B. and M.M. Tabekhia. Changes in Mineral Elements and Phytic Acid Contents During Cooking in Three California Rice Varieties. Journal of Food Science 44(2): 619-621, 1979

188. Recommended Daily Dietary Allowances, Revised 1973. Nutrition Today, 9:20-21, March-April, 1974

189. Goodhart, Robert S. and Maurice E. Shills. Modern Nutrition in Health and Disease. Philadelphia: Lea and Febiger, 1980

190. Bogert, L. Jean. Nutrition and Physical Fitness. Eighth Edition. Philadelphia: W.B. Saunders Company, page 154

191. Iron in Enriched Wheat Flour, Farina, Bread, Buns, and Rolls. Journal of the American Medical Association 220: 855-859, May 8, 1972

192. Murray, M.J. et al. The Adverse Effect of Iron Repletion on the Course of Certain Infections. British Medical Journal 1:1113-1115, October 21, 1978

193. Letcher, Robert L., M.D. Direct Relationship Between Blood Pressure and Blood Viscosity in Normal and Hypertensive Subjects. American Journal of Medicine 70(6):1195-1202, June, 1981

194. Bailey, M.J. et al. Preoperative Haemoglobin as Predictor of Outcome of Diabetic Amputations. Lancet 2:168-170, July 28, 1979

195. Norman, Colin. Iron Enrichment. Nutrition Today, November-December, 1973, page 8-16

196. Butterworth, C.E. Jr. MD Iron "Undercontamination"? Journal of the American Medical Association 220(4):581-582, April 24, 1972

197. Magnesium: Control Over Cell Processes? Science News 108(21):326, November 22, 1975

198. Anderson, Bonnie M. M.Sc. The Iron and Zinc Status of Long-Term Vegetarian Women. American Journal of Clinical Nutrition 34:1042-1048, June, 1981

199. Murphy, Elizabeth W. Provisional Tables on the Zinc Content of Foods. Journal of the American Dietetic Association 66(4):345-355, April, 1975

200. Mirkin, Gabe. Why Seasoned Athletes Succumb to Chronic Fatigue. Washington Post, March 11, 1976

201. Campbell, T. Colin. The Web of Hunger. Natural History Magazine 90(5):12-16, May, 1981

202. Holmes, G. Worchestershire Sauce and the Kidneys. British Medical Journal 2:252, July 24, 1971

203. Murphy, K.J. Sauce, Spices, and the Kidney. British Medical Journal 3:770, September 25, 1971

204. Worchestershire Sauce and the Kidney. The Lancet 2:913, October 3, 1971

205. Olney, John W. M.D. Status of Monosodium Glutamate Revisited. American Journal of Clinical Nutrition 26:683-685, July, 1973

206. Ghadimi, H. M.D. Reply to Dr. Olney, American Journal of Clinical Nutrition 26:686, July, 1973

207. White, Ellen Gould. Testimonies for the Church, Volume 4, Mountain View, California: Pacific Press Publishing Association, 1948, page 141

208. White, Ellen Gould. Counsels on Health, Mountain View, California: Pacific Press Publishing Association, 1951, page 114

209. White, Ellen Gould. Ministry of Healing. Mountain View, California: Pacific Press Publishing Association, 1909, page 305

210. Ibid, page 335

211. White, Ellen Gould. Testimonies for the Church, Volume 3 Mountain View, California: Pacific Press Publishing Association, 1948, page 488

212. Ibid, Page 136

213. Glatzel, H. and M. Ruberg-Schweer. Regional Influence on Cutaneous Blood Flow Effected by Oral Spice Intake. Nutritio et Dieta (Basel) 10:194-214, 1968

214. Solanke, Toriola. The Effect of Red Pepper (Capsicum fructescens) on Gastric Acid Secretion. Journal of Surgical Research 15:385-390, December, 1973

215. MacDonald, W.C. Histological Effect of Certain Pickles on the Human Gastric Mucosa. Canadian Medical Association Journal 96:1521, June 10, 1967

216. Thrash, Agatha Moody, M.D. Eat for Strength. Seale, Alabama: Yuchi Pines Institute

217. Gies, William J. Ph.D. Some Objections to the Use of Alum Baking Powder. Journal of the American Medical Association 57:816-817, September 2, 1911

218. Krantz, John C. Jr. Ph.D. The Pharmacological Principles of Medical Practice. Maryland Psychiatric Research Center, Box 3235, Baltimore, Maryland 21228

219. MacNeal, Herbert P. M.D. Valuable Notes on a Hot Subject. Resident and Staff Physician 27(4):89-92, April, 1981

220. Highland, Joseph and Marcia Fine. Malignant Neglect. New York: Alfred Knopf. 1979, page 239

221. Hidden Dangers in the Bread You Eat. Philadelphian Institute, Inc.

222. Kropf, William M.D. and Milton Houben. Harmful Food Additives. Port Washington, New York: Ashley Books, 1981

223. MacNeal, Herbert P. M.D. Valuable Notes on a Hot Subject. Resident and Staff Physician 27(4):89-92, April, 1981

224. Pathak, J.D. and Pai, M.L. Gastric Response, Digestion, and Evacuation Time of Some Vegetarian Foods. Indian Journal of Medical Research 42:43-49, January, 1954

225. Delire, M. et al. Circulating Immune Complexes in Infants Fed on Cow's Milk. Nature 272:632, April 13, 1978

226. Solanine Poisoning from Potatoes. British Medical Journal 1:1264, April 23, 1960

227. Jaffe, W.G. Toxicity of Raw Kidney Beans. Experientia 5:81, 1949

228. White, Ellen Gould. Counsels on Diet and foods. Takoma Park, Washington D.C.: Review and Herald Publishing Association, 1946, page 95

229. How to Keep Cool. Science News 22:50-51, July 23, 1932

230. Robinson, Dores Eugene. The Story of Our Health Message. Nashville, Tennessee: Southern Publishing Association, 1965, page 58

231. Burrows, Harold. Biological Actions of Sex Hormones. Second Edition, 1949. Cambridge at the University Press, page 304

232. Planas, Antonio T. M.D. Chlorpropamine-Induced Pure RBC Aplasia. Archives of Internal Medicine 140:707-708, 1980

233. Gill, M. John M.D. et al. Hypoglycemic Coma, Jaundice, and Pure RBC Aplasia Following Chlorpropamide Therapy. Archives of Internal Medicine 140:714-715, 1980

234. Kay, R.M. Ph.D. Food Form, Postprandial Glycemia and Satiety. American Journal of Clinical Nutrition 31:738-741, May, 1978

235. Wolf, H.J. and H. Priess. Experiences with Fat Free Diet in Diabetes Mellitus. Deutsche Medizinische Wochenschrift 81:514-551, April 6, 1956

236. Jenkins, David J.A. M.D. Diabetes and Hyperlipidemia: Dietary Implications of Treatment with Fiber. Practical Cardiology 6(11):123-134, October, 1980

237. Schauberger, Gertraud, et al. Exchange of Carbohydrates According to Their Effect on Blood Glucose. Diabetes 26: 415, 1977

238. Jenkins, D.J.A. Bioavailability to Man of Carbohydrate in Foods. Proceedings of the Nutrition Society 39:11A, 1980

239. Durin, J.V.G.A. How Much Food Does Man Require? Nature 242:418, April 6, 1973

240. Johnson, Anita. Unnecessary Chemicals. Enviroment 20(2): 7, March, 1978

241. White, Ellen Gould. Testimonies for the Church, Volume 2, Mountain View, California: Pacific Press Publishing Association, 1948, page 61

242. White, Ellen G. Education. Mountain View, California: Pacific Press Publishing Association, 1952, page 257

243. Grimes, D.S. and C. Gordon. Satiety Value of Wholemeal and White Bread. The Lancet 2:106, July 8, 1978

244. Advising Patients about Fad Diets. Patient Care, June 1, 1976, page 94

245. White, Ellen Gould. Testimonies for the Church, Volume 5, Mountain View, California: Pacific Press Publishing Association, 1948, page 264

246. Romans 12:1, 2

247. Kylen, Anne M. and Rolland M. McCready. Nutrients in Seeds and Sprouts of Alfalfa, Lentils, Mung Beans, and Soybeans. Journal of Food Science 40:1008-1009, 1975

248. White, Ellen Gould. Counsels on Diet and Foods. Takoma Park, Washington D.C.: Review and Herald Publishing Association, 1946, page 322

249. Olney, John W. and Oi-Lan Ho. Brain Damage in Infant Mice Following Oral Intake of Glutamate, Aspartate or Cystine. Nature 227:609, 1970

INDEX

Abdominal pain 94
Acid, blood 102
Acid, stomach 90
Acid-base balance 71
Acid condition 35
Acne 107
Additives 15
Additives, Hazard factors of 82
Adrenalin 99
Adrenals 99, 109
Advertising, Television 25
Aflatoxins 56
Aging 5, 46
Aging, accelerated 105, 109
Aging pigment 66
Akikuyu 20
Alcohol 6, 112
Alcohols 33
Aldehydes 33
Alertness 9
Alkali resistant thermostable factor 69
Alkaloid group 25
Alkaloids, toxic 127
Allergic Reactions 82, 83
Allergies 80, 82, 92, 110, 131
Aluminum 76
Alzheimer's Disease 81
Amaranth 82
American Diabetes Association 105
Amines 33
Amino acid pool 54
Amino acids 4, 5, 22, 35, 51, 52, 92, 93
Ammonia 6, 52
Amylase 34
Andean Indian 2
Androgens 100
Anemias 65
Anemia 21, 41, 69, 106
Anesthesia 6
Anesthetic 43
Angel's food 14
Animal disease 3
Animal kingdom i
Animal products ii, 20
Animal protein 3
Antibiotics 62
Antibodies 22, 55, 58, 92

Antinutrition 25
Antinutritional factors 5
Antioxidants 6, 66
Antioxidant controls 46
Antitoxic 35
Appendicitis 41, 109
Appendix 91, 92
Appetite 11, 14, 54, 58, 63, 88, 100, 121
Appetite control 111, 115
Appetite, exercise curbs 122
Arteries 35
Arthritis 56, 118
Asthma 132
Athletes 34, 121
Atherosclerosis 30, 41, 47, 65
Avidin 65

Babies, healthier 127
Baby foods 83, 84
Bacteria 6, 8, 57
Bad breath 94
Baking powder 74, 81
Baking soda 74, 81
Basic food groups 11, 12
Bates, Captain Joseph 98
Beef 8
Beef protein 7
Behaviour 21
Beriberi 63
Beta-endorphins 59
Between meals, eating 81
Beverages with meals, 115
BHA, 82
BHT, 82
Bile Acids, 8
Bile Salts, 49
"Binge" eating, 122
Biochemical Systems, 20
Biotin, sources of, 65
Birth defects 128
Birth weight, high 108
Bitter flavors 25
Bladder cancer 84
Bladder tumors 41
"Blind Loop Syndrome" 62
Blood chemistries 2, 7
Blood clot 52

Blood clotting 66, 71
Blood destruction 75
Blood formation 69
Blood pressure 37, 41, 73, 100, 118
Blood sugar 39, 65, 99, 108, 109, 110, 112, 115
Blood vessel integrity 65
Blurred vision 63
BMR, athletes 98
BMR, starvation 98
Body regulators 21
Bone loss 53
Bone marrow 7
Bone marrow, depression 75
Botulism 31
Bowel cancer 8
Bowlegs 66
Brain 107
Brain, energy utilization 53
Brain proteins 59
Breakfast 23, 120
Breakfast cereals 25
Breakfast, sample 23
Breast cancer 8, 13
Breast fed infants 68
Breast feeding 66, 109, 132
Breast milk 48, 73, 131
Broken bones 73
Bronchial irritations 29
Buffers 23
Building nutrients 21
Denis Burkett 39
Burning, skin 110
Burns 21
Butchers 6

Cadmium 65
Caffeinated beverages 20
Caffeine 56, 90, 112, 114, 119, 127
Caffeine, medicines containing 113
Cahill, Dr. George 105
Calcium 71, 73
Calcium excretion 53
Calcium metabolism 66
Calcium pump 92
Calcium toxicity 73
Caloric density 68

Caloric requirements 34
Calories, fast walking 34
Calories per gram 37
Calories used per minute 34
Cancer i, 6, 8, 9, 13, 30, 41, 46, 61, 63,
    67, 82, 83, 92, 118
Cancer age 114
Cancer, breast 102
Cancer, cervix 102
Cancer, colon 39
Cancer, Growth of 48
Cancer producing chemical 46
Cancer, stomach, 79
Canning, 31
Caramel, 83
Carbohydrates, yield of glucose, 98
Carious teeth, 73
Carrier System, 36, 91
Carrageenan, 83
Carver, George Washington, 64
Catalysts, 97
Cats 9
Celiac disease 62
Cell turnover 6
Cellulose 39
Central nervous system 65, 80
Cereals, ready-to-eat 23
Charcoal grilled meat 46
Cheerfulness 63
Chemical additive 82
Chemical warfare 22
Chemotaxis 40
Chest pain 84
Chewing 62, 88, 93, 113
Chewing well 68
Child abuse 4
Childbirth 69
Childhood diet 131
Chilling 37, 84
Chilling of the extremities 75, 129
Chinese Coolie 2, 16
Chinese restaurant syndrome 80
Chocolate 79, 119
Chlorinated water 63
Cholera 6
Cholesterol 2, 44, 65, 110, 111
Cholesterol levels 47
Choline sources 55
Chromosome breakage 80
Church trials 19
Circadian rhythm 128
Cirrhosis 4
Clothing, healthful 102
Coffee, substitutes 112
Cold, common 66
Colic, infantile 132
Colitis 83
Colon 92
Colon, bacterial flora 134
Colon, health 36
Colorings 15
Common cold 75
Complex carbohydrates 33, 37
Compost 29
Compulsive thoughts 110
Concentration, poor 109
Confusion 109
Constipation 39, 93, 100, 109
Convenience foods 5
Convulsions 65
Cookbooks 23

Corn 28
Coronary heart disease 13, 22
Coronary heart attacks 37
Cortisol 99
Cortisone 99
Cosmetics 1
Counsels on Diet and Foods 23
Cramps 83
Crash diets 53
Cravings 20, 33, 87, 110, 119, 122, 127
Cravings, Causes of 124
Creatinine 7
Creator i, 2, 12, 54, 59, 71, 94, 97, 117,
    121, 123, 131, 132
Cretinism 101
Crohn's Disease 62
Cyclamates 36
Cysticercosis 6

Dairy Council 3
Dairy industries 8
Dairy milk 73, 131
Dairy products 111
Davidson Dr. Jack 106
Davis, Dr. Donald 39
Degenerative disease, 2, 3, 13, 14, 22
    35, 105, 111
Degenerative processes 29
Dehydrating foods 115
Dehydration 87
Dehydration, chronic 115
Dementia 64
Depression 109
Dermatitis 41, 64
Dental caries 109
Detoxification 94
Dextrins 34
Diabetes 8, 37, 40, 41, 105, 106, 109, 111,
    118
Diabetes, adult onset, 108
Diabetes, Juvenile, 108
Diabetes, Recovery, 108
Diabetes, Viral Triggering, 106
Diabetics, 107
Diarrhea, 64, 66, 84, 94, 100
Diet, unpalatable, 17
Diet, well balanced, 53
Diffusion 91
Digestion 21, 62, 88, 93
Diglycerides 83
Dinners 120
Disaccharides, 34
Discernment, 110
Disposition, sour, 19
Diuretics, 87
Diverticulosis, 39
Divine help, 119
(DNA) Deoxyribonuclic acid, 6
Dogs 3, 9
Dopamine 100
Drinking water 6
Drug addicts 6
Drugs 6, 62, 90
Duodenal ulcer 41, 81
Duodenum 90
Eat For Strength 23, 37, 111, 112
Eating between meals 90, 93, 122
Eating errors 121
Eating habits 68
Eating slowly 68
Ecology 14

Economy 3, 7, 8, 9, 16, 37
EDTA 83
Eggs 8
"Egg White Injury" 65
Electroshock therapy 110
Emotional instability 2
Emotional stability 21
Emotions, balanced 14
Empty calories 58
Emulsified peanut butter 25
Emulsions 44
Encephalitis 76
Endurance 16
Enema, cold 100
Energy 21, 35, 98
Energy used 119
Encephalins 59
Enriched bread 74
Enzymes 21, 30, 33, 97
Eskimo 106
Essential foods 12
Essential nutrients 12
Estrogen, foods low in 102
Estrogen therapy 76
Estrogens 8, 100
Eucalyptus oil 80
Evening meals 122
Evolution, Theory of 97
Exercise 7, 37, 75, 113, 115
Extravagant food bill 1

Fad diets 121
Failure to thrive 4
Farming, Methods of 27
Fast 102, 108
Fast 7
Fasting 102, 108
Fat diet 13
Fat digestion 93
Fatigue 75, 77, 82
Fat metabolism 35
Fats 43
Fats, caloric content 45
Fats, Proportion of 44
Fats, Saturation of 45
Fats, Yield of glucose 98
Fatty acids, cis 46
Fatty acids, trans 46
Favism 56
Fecal flora 95
Feeding, don'ts for 135
Fermentation 46, 81, 90, 94
Fermentation products 33
Fermented foods 122
Fermented products 114
Fertility 66
Fertilizers, commercial 29
Fiber diet, high 39
Fibers, plant 36
Fibrin 52
Fingernails, spotted 76
Flavorings 15
"Fleshpots of Egypt" 19
Fletcher, Horace 19
Flood, The 7, 13
Fluid retention 71
Fluids, inter-cellular 23
Food additives 81
Food additives, twenty worst 82
Food consumed 13
Food faddism 20

Food habits 22
Food, rich 20
Food, calming 79
Foods, Combination of 62
Foods, concentrated 68
Foods, depressing 79
Food sensitivities 111, 134
Food shortages 12
Food supplements 6
Food, Nutritive effects of 56
Foods, Pharmacologic effects of 56
Foods, sedative 79
Foods, stimulating 79
Foods, Varieties of at one meal 70
Forgetfulness 109
Fossilized ferns 13
Framingham Study 47
Free radicals 66
Freezing foods 66
Fructose 33
Frying 46, 66

Galactose 33
Gallbladder 73, 93
Gallbladder disease 107
Gallstones 41
Gas formation 88
Gas fuel 29
Gas, intestinal 94
Gastritis 81
Gastrointestinal tract 22, 58
General adaptation syndrome 109
Generation age 13, 108
Genetic damage 84
Genetic effects 83
Gums 83
Giardiasis 62
Glandular stimulation 107
Glucagon 93
Glucocorticoids 99
Glycogen 36, 107
Glucose 33, 107
Glucose pump 92
Glucose Tolerance Test 110
Gluten-Free Diet 37
Goiter 28, 76
Gout 7, 41, 66, 118
Goiter Belts 28
Gout 7, 41, 66, 118
Grady Hospital 108
Graham Sylvestor 39
Grains, Cooking of 36, 76, 134
Growth acceleration 107
Growth hormones 107
Growth rates 14, 108

Habits 25, 131
Hardinge 21
Headache 29, 33, 63, 84, 94, 110, 115
Health conditioning centers 47
Health reform 12
Heart attacks 8
Heart beat, fast 110
Heartburn 90
Heart defects 82
Heart disease 9, 39, 47
Heart palpitation 82
Heart valves 73
Heavenly Father 18
Hemodialysis 76
Hemoglobin 2, 53, 55, 57, 65, 74

Hemoglobin, Ideal for women 74
Hemoglobin readings 110
Hemorrhoids 39, 110
Hepatitis A 6
Herbert, Dr. Victor 69
Herbs 79
Hiatus hernia 90
Hinder 2
Histamine 100
Home economics 11
Hormones, steroid 65
Human history 132
Human milk, Nutrient content of 132
Hunger 23, 87, 88, 123
Hunzakuts 20
Hydrochloric acid 94
Hydroponic 27
Hydroxylated lecithin 83
Hyperactive 4
Hyperactivity in children 82
Hypertension 80
Hyperthyroidism 100
Hypoglycemic syndrome 109, 111
Hypoglycemic syndrome, Questions
   about 113
Hypothyroidism 100

Impatience 19
Indecisiveness 109
Infant feeding 133
Infant formulas 66
Infantile eczema 132
Infections 55, 63, 65
Infections, host defense against 74
Infertility 41
Influenza 75, 106
Influenza pandemic 41
Insulin 39, 50, 76, 93, 94
Intellectual activity 15
Intemperate 119
Intestinal gas 92
Intestinal problems 83
Iodine 76
IQ, baby's 128
IQ, breast fed infants 131
Iron 65, 74, 92, 133, 134
Iron absorption 41, 66
Iron deficiency 74
Iron intake, increased 76
Iron overload 74
Irritable 110
Itching 63

John the Baptist 14
Joints 35, 73
Judgmental activities 110
Junk foods 5
Juvenile diabetes 105, 108

Kellogg, John Harvey 19
Ketone bodies 35
Keys, Ancel 21
Kidneys 2, 22, 35, 39, 52, 58, 73, 75, 80,
   83, 107, 109, 121
Kidney stones 7, 66, 80
Kreb's Cycle 35
Kwashiorkor 59

Laboratory results, ideal 110
Lactose deficiency 94
Lactic acid 35, 83

Lactose 34, 94
Lactose intolerance 56, 69
Latins 22
Leafy vegetables 20, 36, 63, 74, 123
Learning 63
Legume-grain combination 22
Length of life 2
Leukemia i, 8
Leukemia, myelogenous 67
Lifespan 7, 13
Lifestyle i, 5, 7
Linoleic acid 47
Lipids 43
Lipofuscin 46, 66
Liver 2, 6, 22, 35, 39, 58, 84, 109, 113, 121
Liver ailments 82
Liver tumors 85
Lunch, sample 123
Lymphatic system 43
Lymphatic leukemia 8

Magnesium 76
Maillard reaction 37
Main dishes 123
Malignancies 40
Malignant growths 82
Malnutrition 19, 23
Maltol dextril 83
Mania 100
Manna 14
Man naturally a vegetarian 7
Marriage, early 109
Masai 20
Mastication 19
Maternal weight gain 127
Maturation, early 108
Maturity onset diabetes 105
Meal planning 11
Mealtimes, regular 111
Meat diet, 1
Meat substitutes 111
Meditating 63
Medical care 9
Medical missionary work 64
Medical practitioners 11
Medical schools 11
Megavitamin therapy 61
Melba toast 112, 134
Memory loss 59
Menarche 108
Menopause 101
Menstrual problems 118
Mental alertness 21
Mental attitude 128
Mental capacity 52
Mental confusion 110
Mental disorders 39
Mental illness 33
Mental dullness 39, 94
Mental efficiency 29
Mental function 9
Mental illness 4, 8, 33
Mental productivity 11
Menu content 122
Metabolism 97
Metal, trace 28
Microwave oven 29
Milk 8
Milk, nut 111
Milk, nutrient content of cow 132
Milk production 132

Milk, soy 111
Milk substitutes 12
Milk-sugar combinations 90
Milling of grains 66
Mind, clearer 1
Mind cure 119
Mineralocorticoids 99
Mineral oil 62
Minerals 71
Mirkin, Dr. Gabe 77
Mitochondria 21
Modified food starch 83
Monoglycerides 83

Monosaccharides, 34
Monosodium glutamate (MSG) 25, 80, 84
Mood swings 107, 110
Mood sensibilities 80
Mortality 41
Mouth 89
Multivitamin preparations 69
Mumps 106
Mumps virus 89
Muscle contraction 21, 71
Muscle relaxation 21
Muscles 73
Mutagenic 14
Mutagenic effects 80
Mutagens 6
Mutations 6
Myoglobin 55

National Cancer Institute 82
National Poultry and Meat Association 3
Natural food of man 1
Nephritis 52
Nerve cell developers 131
Nerve impulses 21
Nerves 35
Nerve transmission 71
Nervous disorders 55
Nervousness 82, 100, 109
Nervous system 21
"Nesting Instinct" 109
Neurosis 100
Nibbling 52
Nicotine 90, 112, 127
Nightmares 109
Nitrates, sodium 84
Norepinephrine 100
Nutrient losses 30
Nutrients, content in food 29
Nutrition, primary rule of 12, 30
"Nutritional Degenerative Disease" 105
Nutritionists 3
Nutrition supplement ii
NUTRITION TODAY, 106

Obesity 1, 2, 41, 118
Obsessions 110
Office workers 16
Oil-free diet 113
Oils 46
Oligosaccharides 34
Oral anti-diabetic agents 115
Oral contraceptives 65
Organic brain disease 76
Organic gardening 28
Orientals 22
Osmosis 91
Osteoporosis 5, 102
Overeating 12, 20, 90, 118

Overeating, cure for 119
Overnutrition 11, 19
Overpopulation 33
Overweight 7, 24, 55, 117, 120
Overweight, cause of 122
Overweight, dangers of 118

Pain 59
Palatability 62
Palatability of food 87
Pancreatitis 41
Pantothenic acid 65
Pastas 7
PBB's (polybrominated biphenyls) 8
Pectins 36
Pellagra 4, 64
Pepsin 94
Peptic ulcer 6
Peristalsis 66, 90, 95
Pernicious anemia 67
Peroxides 46
Phagocytic index 24
Phagocytosis 40
Phenacetin 7
Phenylketonuria 56
Phenylethylanine 100
Phospholipids 44
Phosphorus 76
Photosynthesis 5, 21
Physical stamina 21
Physiologist 1
Phytase 73
Phytates 66
Phytic acid 73
Pigmentation of skin 99
Pima Indians 106
Pituitary 37
Pneumonia 106
Polysaccharides 34
Polysorbate 84
Poor families 12
Posture 75
Poultry 8
Potatoes 2
Potato chips 24
Poverty 1
Prayer, 121
Praying 63
Pregnancy diet 127
Pregnancy, marital relations during 128
Pregnant women 16
Prenatal care 128
Pressor amines 100
Pritikin, Nathan 47
Processed foods 82
Propylene glycol alginate 84
Propyl gallate 84
Prostate 102
Protein 3, 51
Protein diet, dehydration and 121
Protein diet, high 22
Protein deficiency 5, 7, 22, 52, 58
Protein digestion 94
Protein, excess 13, 52
Protein foods 33
Protein intake, low 52
Protein requirements of 55
Protein sparing 35, 37
Protein, Overeating of 35
Proteins, yield of glucose 98
Psychotic 4

Puberty, earlier 107
Purines 7, 119
Purine content 58

Rancidity 37
Raw diet 4
RDA (Recommended Daily Allowance) 5
Red dye 84
Red II dye 36, 82
Reducing diet 120
Reducing diet, sample 125
Refining 15
Religious life 15
Rennin 94
Restlessness 33, 82
Rheumatoid arthritis 40, 67
Rich diet 2
Rickets 66
RNA (Ribonucleic acid) 6
Runners, long distance 16
Saccharin 41, 84
Salivary glands 89
Salmonellosis 6
Salt, free use of 122
Satiety 46
Satiety value 121
Scalp symptoms 110
Scarlet fever 106
Schizophrenia 4
School dropout 109
Scurvey 65
Seafood 6
Seasonings 79
Sedentary workers 16
Seizures 59
Selenium 76
Self-control 11, 117, 119
Selye, Hans 109
Senility 76
Senna tea 100
Sense of well-being 69
Serotonin 55, 100
Seventh-day Adventist ii, 2, 12
Seventh-day Adventist women 76
Sex hormones 100
Sexual development 109
Sexual maturity 13
Shellfish 6
Simple diet 6, 14
Simple fare 1
Simplicity 16
Sin, dominion 119
Sirloin steak 4
Sitz bath 102
Skin 73
Skin disease 39
Skin irritations 83
Skin rashes 83
Skin, scaling of 63
Sleep 123
Sleep, before midnight 114
Small intestine 91
Smell 63
Smog 66
Smokers 7
Smoking 3
Social occasions 114
Sodium 73
Sodium erythrobate 84
Sodium pump 71, 92
Soil, poor 27

Solanine 56, 94
Soy milk 113
Soy milk, commercial 111
Soy sauce 79
Soybean protein 1
Spaghetti 7
Specific dynamic action 22
Spices 79
Sprouting 125
Sprouting, method of 126
Sprue 62
Starch, cooking of 36
Starvation 98
Starvation diet 5
Sterility 118
Sterols 48
Sterols, plant 48, 101
Stillman Diet 53
Stomach 80, 90
Stomach acids 81
Stomach, emptying time of 90, 93
Stomach irritants 114, 122
Stomach, sour 19
Stare, Dr. 21
Stoves, kitchen 29
Strength 29, 98
Streptococcal sore throat 55
Stress 62, 113
Stressful lifestyle 12
Stroke 9, 37
Sucrose 39
Sudden death 65
Sudden Infant Death Syndrome 132
Suicidal tendencies 109
Sugar 92, 93, 106
Sugar problems 39
Sugar substitutes 118
Sweating 84, 87
Sugar, Sweetness of 35
Sweets 111
Summer 16
Sunshine 75
Supper 115
Supplements 6
Tannin 85
Tarahumara Indians 5, 16
Taste 63

Taste buds, 24, 89
Tea, substitutes, 112
Teenage rebellion, 109
Teeth 8, 89, 107
Teether 134
Temper 24
Temperance 19
Temptation 119, 122
Tempted, help for 119
Thanksgiving 54, 95
Theobromine 79
Theophyllin 79
Thiaminase 5
Thiourea 100
Thirst 87
Thymidine 6
Thyroid 37, 76, 100
Thyroid hormone 55
Tobacco 68
Tomato 28
Tongue 89
Tongue, sore 55
Tonsils 91
Tooth decay 39
Toxic overload of protein 57
Toxic properties of foods 94
Toxic symptoms 56
Toxic waste 22
Toxins 33
Trichinosis 6
Triglycerides 36, 44, 50, 110
Tryptamine 100
Tryptophan, sources of 64
Tuskegee Institute 64
Two-meal plan 111, 133
Typhoid 6
Tyramine 100
Ulcerative colitis 62, 67
Undernutrition 11
Undernutrition, selective 20
Underweight 63, 125
Unleavened bread 66
Uric acid 2, 17
Urinary tract infections 107
Urine, color of 87
U.S. Department of Agriculture 4
Vaginal infections 107

Variation of nutrients in foods 27
Variety of foods 122
Vegan 3, 4, 8, 68, 69
Vegan Society 7
Vegetarian women 102
Vibriosis 6
Vinegar 81
Viral infections 75
Viruses 6
Vitamin B-1 (Thiamine) 63
Vitamin B-2 (Riboflavin) 63
Vitamin B-6 (Pyridoxine) 65
Vitamin B-6, Sources of 65
Vitamin B-12 61, 62, 63, 66, 92
Vitamin B-12, anti-breakdown
    products 69
Vitamin C 6, 65
Vitamin D 66
Vitamin E (Tocopherol) 66
Vitamins 61
Vitamins, Losses of 62
Vitamins, pharmacodynamic effect 61
Voice, high-pitched 87
Vomiting 94
Walking 34, 114
Weakness 113
Weaning 134
Weight 2
Weight calculation 118
Weight control 56, 104
Weight, ideal 117
Weight loss diets 53
Weight reduction 108, 119, 122
White blood cell counts 7
White blood cells 39
White, Paul Dudley 47
Will power 119, 122, 123
Wine 19
Wound healing 65, 69, 76, 107
Yemenite Jews 39, 106
Young people, problems of 67
Yuchi Pines Institute ii, 47
Yudkin, John 41
Zinc 76
Zinc absorption 66
Zwiebach 82

Other Books by the Drs. Thrash...

Animal Connection–according to the U. S. Department of Agriculture, there is no fowl or livestock anywhere that can be guaranteed disease-free. Pets also can be carriers of lethal ailments. Find out how to protect yourself. $6.95 US

Nutrition for Vegetarians–the nutrition guide for all, vegetarian or non-vegetarian! Discussion of food groups, supplements, facts and fallacies.
$14.95 US

Eat for Strength Cookbook–completely vegetarian, and oil-free! Tasty, appealing and very low fat. Also, menus and meal planners included. $8.95 US

Food Allergies Made Simple–an interesting and thorough handling of this controversial subject. How to determine a sensitivity, variety for a new diet, etc. $4.95 US

Diabetes & the Hypoglycemic Syndrome–many new facts are continually coming to light concerning the onset and control of diabetes, including a different look at the complete diet (not just sugar). The Drs. Thrash have put current information with nearly 40 years of medical practice to culminate in this book. $14.95 US

Fatigue: Causes, Prevention & Treatment–fatigue is said to be one of the most common complaints heard in physicians' offices in the United States today! This book is a complete manual, covering causes, treatments and prevention all natural! $4.95 US

Home Remedies–the complete How-To for natural treatment, specializing in water- (or hydro-) therapy. Also, diagnosis, massage, charcoal, garlic and other herbal therapies, exercises for healing, and more! If you can only afford one book for your family's health problems, this is the one! Quoted from by other books, including *Doctor's Book of Home Remedies*. Get the full text! $14.95 US

Natural Remedies
More Natural Remedies–the manuals that list nearly 100 diseases and practical prevention and treatment of each. From acne to tennis elbow, these straight-forward books list the disease, then the treatment. Differs from *Home Remedies* in size and scope, and focuses specifically on the disease and treatments, and not so much the methods. $6.95 ea. US

Rx: Charcoal–charcoal is a most amazing substance! Takes up poisons, and is non-toxic, with no side effects. Find out how to use it, including venomous bites, stings, detox, poison control, stomach upset, "food poisoning", and much more. A must for every home. $6.95 US

Natural Healthcare for Your Child–similar to *Natural* and *More Natural Remedies*, except with a focus on children's diseases. Includes prenatal care and diagnosis. $9.95

Also, booklets on: *Fertility, Contraception and Abortion*; *Poison with a Capital C* (caffeine); *The Prostate*; and a *Simple Home Remedies* manual, all $3.00 each, US

All prices are in US dollars, and are subject to change. Contact NewLifestyle Books for current prices and shipping charges.

NewLifestyle Books, Seale, AL 36875 (334/855-4708 or 800/542-5695)